OXFORD MEDICAL PUBLICATIONS

The Anaesthetic *Aide-Mémoire*

The Anaesthetic
Aide-Mémoire

JOHN URQUHART

Oxford   New York   Tokyo

OXFORD UNIVERSITY PRESS

1996

Oxford University Press, Walton Street Oxford OX2 6DP

Oxford   New York
Athens   Auckland   Bangkok   Bombay
Calcutta   Cape Town   Dar es Salaam   Delhi
Florence   Hong Kong   Istanbul   Karachi
Kuala Lumpur   Madras   Madrid   Melbourne
Mexico City   Nairobi   Paris   Singapore
Taipei   Tokyo   Toronto
and associated companies in
Berlin   Ibadan

Oxford is a trade mark of Oxford University Press

Published in the United States
by Oxford University Press Inc., New York

© John Urquhart 1996

A catalogue record for this book is available from the British Library

Library of Congress Cataloging in Publication Data
(Data available)

ISBN 0 19 262690 6

Typeset by Hewer Text Composition Services, Edinburgh

Printed in Great Britain by The Bath Press, Somerset

Contents

Introduction and acknowledgements

The *Anaesthetic Aide-Mémoire* is a compilation of lists and diagrams intended as a ready reference for anaesthetists in training and for consultants in anaesthesia. It is not, and is not meant to be, a definitive pocket textbook of anaesthesia; it is for reference when a fact, statistic or formula eludes the memory. It is also an aid to teaching.

It covers lists, numerical data, physiological and pharmacological formulae, information on illnesses pertaining to anaesthesia, data on equipment, clinical measurement and intensive care management. It includes recent recommendations by the Royal College of Anaesthetists and the Association of Anaesthetists of Great Britain and Ireland, on safety, audit and other postgraduate matters. It does not include anatomy; there are textbooks on anatomy for anaesthetists. It does not deal with the derivations of physiological and pharmacological equations. Neither is it a pharmacopoeia. This book is intended for anaesthetists who have passed that stage, but who merely want to be reminded of a particular equation or formula prior to using it clinically, or asking a junior to produce it in a practice exam.

It will also be useful for candidates for the FRCA Examination, who will already understand the physiology and pharmacology but who need their memory jogged on occasion.

I am indebted to the following people for their help and for reading specific areas of the manuscript that are of interest to them.

Dr. Karen Simpson, for reading and correcting the entire manuscript, a task performed with meticulous attention to detail.
Mr. Andrew Malyon, the only surgeon to have been allowed near the manuscript, for his ideas on the view from beyond the blood brain barrier.
Dr. Mark Blunt, for reading the Practical Anaesthesia section, and for suggestions on that. Dr. John Scully, for reading the Audit and Admin section, and for many typically mature suggestions.
Dr. Nilufer Mahmood, for reading the Pharmacology and Stats section. Dr. Cathy Roud Mayne, for reading and advising on the longest section - Preop and Preparation. Dr. Jacky Gedney, for reading the sections on ITU, Resus and Critical Incident Management. Dr. Roger Garforth, for reading the

Physiology section. Dr. David Scott, for advice on connective tissue disease. Finally, Dr. Saxon Ridley, for advice on the matter of statistics and measurement.

John Urquhart

Anaesthetic Department
Norfolk & Norwich Hospital
Brunswick Road
Norwich
February 1996

Thinking and teaching

WISDOM

Life is too short to drink flat tonic

John Winn

On education:

For most men it remains true and even obvious that for the best education a complete general training in fields other than those of their future calling brings about a richer result.

Bill's observation; that a person may be educated beyond their intelligence.

On anaesthesia and medicine:

You are more likely to die on the first day of your life than on any other than your last

Professor John Davis

If the surgeon cuts a vessel and knows the name of that vessel, the situation is serious; if the anaesthetist knows the name of that vessel, the situation is irretrievable

Dr M Morgan

III: at a cardiac arrest the first procedure is to take your own pulse
IV: the patient is the one with the disease
VII: there is no body cavity that cannot be reached with a 14g needle and a good strong arm
X: if you don't take a temperature you can't find a fever
XIII: the delivery of medical care is to do as much nothing as possible

Samuel Shem

Smith's law of pharmacology:
If a drug is lipid soluble, it will be absorbed orally, it will cross the blood brain barrier and the placenta, it will be reabsorbed by the kidneys and will therefore be metabolised and conjugated.

The Anaesthetic Aide-Mémoire

If a drug is water soluble, it will not be absorbed orally, it will not cross the blood brain barrier or the placenta, and will be filtered by the kidneys.

Mac's law: anaesthesia is easy. As long as the blood is going round and round, and the air is going in and out, the worst that can happen is that the patient will wake up.

Extremes of opinion and practice are the posts that mark out the path of medical progress.

Always remember that the kit you are using was made by the lowest bidder.

Jowitt's law: at night, if alone, if in trouble, with private cases, use scoline.

Salmon's law: when anaesthetising children, the sum of the pulse rate of the child and the anaesthetist will always equal 150.

Winn's modification: that a coefficient be applied to Salmon's law where the more junior and frightened the anaesthetist the greater is that coefficient

Aunty Gwen's rule: wait until you see upper limb flexion before you take the tube out and you won't see laryngospasm

Muscle relaxants do not make the hole bigger, they do not relax bone, they do not decompress bowel, they do not give a surgeon judgement, and they do not relax fat.

On making it count:

Sutton's law: Sutton, an american bank robber, was asked as he was about to be hanged, why he robbed banks. "Because that's where the money is".

Cullen's law: rugby is a game of possession, but mostly of territory; in order to win, any incursion beyond the enemy's 22 metre line must result in the scoring of points.

On sex:

The Urquhart-Malyon law: the innuendo implies the deed.

On intensive care:

Thorp's maxim of intensive care: if a patient isn't going forwards, he's going backwards.

The management of an intensive care patient is characterised by an initial period when resuscitation calls for administration of large quantities of fluid, and a subsequent period when it has to be retrieved.

The time to do a laparotomy is when you first think of it.

On management:

Political handling of a crisis: (after Hacker)
Stage 1: there isn't going to be a problem.
Stage 2: there might be a problem, but there isn't anything we would be able to do about it.
Stage 3: there is a problem, but it would be inappropriate for us to do anything about it.
Stage 4: there was a problem, we might have been able to do something, but the time has passed.

Barbara Morgan on obstetrics:

General anaesthesia for Caesarean Section for fetal distress kills mothers who had nothing wrong with them.

The anaesthetist is there to look after the mother: the paediatrician is there to look after the baby: the obstetrician is there to look after himself.

The decision regarding surgery is the obstetrician's. The anaesthesia must be left to the anaesthetist.

You can take an orthopaedic surgeon to slaughter, but you can't make him think.

Dr. Phil Keep

SEVENTEEN RULES OF LECTURING

Don't apologise for having insufficient time.
Don't apologise for the subject you're presenting.
Don't turn your back on the audience.
Don't use grubby, faded or handwritten visual aids.
Don't obstruct the view of the screen, with yourself or the projector.
Don't use abbreviations or acronyms without explaining them.
Don't use annoying mannerisms.
Don't invite students to write it down and then snatch the overhead away.
Don't wave the laser pointer around the screen or the audience.

Do make sure you know where everything is in the lecture theatre before you start.
Do introduce yourself.
Do say at the beginning what you are going to talk about - and what you aren't.
Do speak up, and to the back of the room.
Do make eye contact.
Do produce a handout, which is intelligible.
Do present a summary at the end.

Never use any of the following words or expressions:
interactive
it's all in the textbooks
group dynamics
learning curve

IN A SURGEON'S GOWN

A nmemonic for describing a pathological condition, its management and treatment.

....Even A Physician May Make Some Strange Clinically Complicated Points, Perhaps

DEFINITION
INCIDENCE, MORBIDITY, MORTALITY
AGE
SEX, RACE
GEOGRAPHIC
ECONOMIC
AETIOLOGY, ASSOCIATIONS
PATHOLOGY
MACROSCOPIC
MICROSCOPIC
STAGING
SPREAD
CLINICAL = MANAGEMENT: Sexy Stephanie Inserts One Diaphragm Tonight
    SYMPTOMS
    SIGNS
    INVESTIGATIONS
    OBSERVATIONS
    DIFFERENTIALS
    TREATMENT: Many Conservative Secretaries Promise Some Nice Favours
        MEDICAL
        CONSERVATIVE
        SURGICAL
        PALLIATIVE
        SOCIAL
        NURSING
        FOLLOW UP
COMPLICATIONS and of treatment
PROGNOSIS
PREVENTION

HOW TO DESCRIBE A DRUG

A nmemonic for the description of any drug or preparation.

Pretty Cute Anaesthetists Can Undo Dresses Regardless Of Displeasure Clearly Covering Sister's Expression In Theatre:

PRESENTATION: Tablets, injection, colour
CHEMICAL NATURE: Draw if appropriate, e.g. volatiles
ACTION: At receptor level
CLASS: E.g. Vaughan Williams
USES: Stress anaesthetic uses but do not omit those that the rest of the world uses the drug for
DOSE: Obvious
ROUTE OF ADMINISTRATION: Again, obvious, but don't guess; for example, alfentanil only has a licence for IV use, whereas fentanyl has a licence for IV and IM
ONSET: Rapid, slow, delayed
DURATION OF ACTION: Short, medium, long; state the half-life if you know it
CONTRAINDICATIONS: Absolute and relative
COMPLICATIONS: These are the serious ones like asystole and agranulocytosis, in contrast to:
SIDE EFFECTS: Which are the trivial ones like nausea and vomiting, but these two (side effects and complications) do overlap
ELIMINATION: Generally hepatic or renal, but remember pulmonary elimination and excretion of drug into breast milk. In general, if a drug is lipid-soluble, it will be absorbed orally, it will cross the BBB and the placenta, it will be reabsorbed by the kidneys and therefore be eliminated by metabolism and conjugation. If a drug is water-soluble, it will not be absorbed orally, will not cross the BBB or placenta, and will be filtered by the kidneys.
INTERACTIONS: With what, and the effect: enhancement of one or other
THE GRAVID UTERUS: See above.

HOW TO HANDLE A CLINICAL NIGHTMARE AT PART 1

1. Can I get out of giving this anaesthetic?
2. Can I get someone else to give this anaesthetic?
3. Can I stall by getting a physician to optimise therapy?
4. If I must give it, can I have a senior colleague present?
5. Can I get out of giving a GA by using a regional or local technique instead?

➡ The penetrating eye injury is not a surgical emergency, and can wait until starved, and even then can often be done under local anaesthesia
➡ #NOFs do not have to be done at 0300 as long as they are done within 48 hours
➡ At the rapid sequence induction, I shall give a predetermined sleep dose of induction agent; at other times I shall titrate to response
➡ At the rapid sequence induction, I shall give a calculated dose of suxamethonium immediately the patient is asleep; at other times I shall first ensure that I can control the airway
➡ If I forget suction at the rapid sequence induction I shall not pass the exam

THE VIEW FROM BEYOND THE BLOOD-BRAIN BARRIER

Or - the dreams of the surgeon in choosing one's anaesthetist. Note immediately that the surgeon always refers to *my* anaesthetist and *my* theatre sister. It is our one remaining delusion, please don't take it away!

If you can satisfy the '4 As' sought at job interviews throughout the country, then most surgeons will have difficulty finding grounds for complaint (although the more determined will always succeed).

Affability: "easy of address, courteous". Life can be so much less stressful if one can turn to the head of the table and exchange a pleasantry rather than a snarl. Surgeons are, of course, always particularly affable, especially when returning to theatre at 3am to redo a microvascular anastomosis on a free flap that isn't quite working.

Availability: "at one's disposal". If a case has to be done, then it sometimes has to be done., and much though we might hate to admit it, the anaesthetist can be indispensable. Excuses like "I'm just off to check through the last six months of *Anaesthesiology* to see if I can find the article on the widget in beer cans" may not wash too well. When we've all grown up and become Consultants, this area does have special financial considerations in the private sector, and can then seem to be less of a problem.

Amiability: "Feeling and inspiring friendliness". Similar to affability. It might come as a shock to think that a surgeon would actually want an anaesthetist as a friend, but this just shows what generous people surgeons are. Once again, stress reduction can be achieved if there is a relaxed and friendly atmosphere in theatre.

Ability: "Having the power to; talented; clever". It gives a surgeon great comfort to know that, in spite of all his or her efforts, the patient will survive the operation in question due to the efforts of the anaesthetist. In particular, surgeons hate patients moving during their operation, and patients trying to help put their own dressings on. If you can prevent this you will be in demand.

PS - Having been adopted by a surgeon, remember (not) to try out some of these old favourite lines :

To the struggling SHO at 2am

> "Does Mr .... know you do it that way?"
> "I thought the appendix was an the right"
> "Anyone got a calendar?"

To the unhappy Registrar on a routine list

> "Your SHO does this operation very well"
> "Are you sure Mr .... is on holiday"
> "I don't think you wanted to do that"
> "When I was Mr ....'s houseman I used to do....."

To the Consultant

> Being (almost) perfect there will be no opportunity to use your razor-like wit at the expense of the consultant.

And Finally,

Remember that when the consultant suddenly says "oh SH-one-T" in the middle of a case the immediate action drills are to put in at least 2 14G cannulae, a central line, cross match 8 units and phone home to say you're going to be late.

Definitions taken from Pocket Oxford Dictionary Fifth edition.

Notes

Fibre		Diam (μm)	V (m/s)
A	α JPS, Motor	12-20	70-120
	β Touch, Pressure	5-12	30-70
	γ Motor - Muscle spindle	3-6	15-30
	δ ~~preganglionic~~ Pain Temp	~~~~ 2-5	12-30
B	Preganglionic Autonomic	<3	3-15
C	Dorsal Root - Pain Temp	0·4-1·2	0·5-2
	Symp Postganglionic	0·3-1·3	0·7-2·3

A + B   myelinated

___

EEG

β - 13-30 - Infants / Frontal

α - 8-10 (rest eyes shut)

Theta - 4-8

δ - <4   normal in kids
                 + asleep.

The preoperative period and preparation for anaesthesia

PREOPERATIVE ASSESSMENT

This is intended to remind the busy anaesthetist of the essential questions and features of examination and preoperative investigation.

HISTORY

PREVIOUS GENERAL ANAESTHETICS
Family History of allergy or adverse reaction. The important ones are malignant hyperpyrexia and suxamethonium apnoea.
PAST MEDICAL HISTORY
General health and systematic review, with especial reference to exercise tolerance, orthopnoea and other indicators of ischaemic heart disease.
Specific questions:

- Coryza or productive cough
- Dyspepsia; if so, is there oesophageal reflux?
- Smokes; anticipate airway irritability in heavy smokers. The other problems associated with tobacco include high carboxyhaemoglobin levels, which impair oxygen carriage; ciliary dysfunction; and increased secretions.
- Bleeding tendencies; easy bruising is a good discriminator
- Drugs
- Allergies

EXAMINATION
TEETH; loose teeth, false teeth, caps or crowns.
MOUTH: for ease of intubation.

Mallampati classification:	Wilson grading (jaw protrusion)
I uvula, complete view	A: Lower incisors beyond upper
II base of uvula only seen	B: Edge-to-edge
III soft palate in view	C: Lower cannot come edge-to-
IV hard palate only	edge. Always difficult.

NECK. for flexion and extension, and for precipitation of vertebro-basilar insufficiency if susceptible.

WEIGHT
CHEST auscultation; blood pressure, heart rate, heart sounds

INVESTIGATIONS

Use a matrix built around Haematology, Chemistry, XRay and Clinical Measurement to remind you:

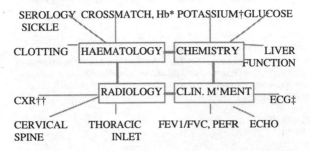

*Haemoglobin should be measured in menstruating women, where there are symptoms of anaemia, and in all over age 55. It is pointless in fit young men.

†Chemistry is indicated in patients on cardiac drugs, the effects of which are modulated by electrolyte derangement, and those on diuretics; these give rise to derangement, especially causing low potassium. Also consider chemistry in all diabetics. Otherwise, restrict to those over 55.

††1979 Royal College of Radiologists; routine Chest XRay is not justified as a preoperative test, but may be desirable in acute respiratory distress, where metastatic disease is suspected, in chronic airways disease where no XRay has been performed in the previous year, and where the possibility of pulmonary tuberculosis exists.

‡ECG is indicated where there is a cardiac history and in symptomatic patients. It should also be performed in the over 50 age group, and in diabetics over 40. There is great value in making comparison with previous ECG recordings.

American Society of Anesthesiologists (ASA) I no illness II mild III incapacitated IV threat to life V moribund; **E** is added to denote emergency

NCEPOD DEGREE OF URGENCY
ELECTIVE: At a time to suit both patient and surgeon
SCHEDULED: Early operation, usually within 3 weeks
URGENT: As soon as possible, usually within 24 hours
EMERGENCY: Immediate, resuscitation simultaneous with operation.

NIL BY MOUTH SOLIDS/LIQUIDS
Adults are traditionally starved 6 hours to solids and 3 hours to liquids.
Children should be starved for shorter periods. The issue becomes
irrelevant in an emergency, although it is valuable to know the duration of
the interval between last meal and trauma or administration of opiates,
since this is more relevant in terms of gastric emptying than the interval
between last meal and induction of anaesthesia.

THROMBOEMBOLIC RISK
PROPHYLAXIS IF INDICATED (see below)

PREMEDICATION
Nothing is so useful as the preoperative visit.
PATIENT'S NORMAL MEDICATION (but not oral hypoglycaemics,
and possibly not monoamine oxidase inhibitors)
NOTHING; EMLA CREAM AND A PARENT; in the under three,
consider augmenting this with oral atropine (0.425 mg or 0.85 mg)
SODIUM CITRATE & H_2 ANTAGONISTS where reflux is a possibility
and a rapid sequence induction is planned
β-AGONISTS; OR β-BLOCKERS? Asthma, or ischaemic heart disease?
FLUID PRELOAD if jaundiced, as prophylaxis against the hepatorenal
syndrome
IV DEXTROSE AND INSULIN in diabetes
OPIATE OR BENZODIAZEPINE for the traditionalist anaesthetist and
the anxious patient - but remember the value of the preoperative visit in
allaying anxiety.

SCORING IN ASSESSMENT

GLASGOW COMA SCALE
Best score = 15; worst 3. A score of 8 is regarded as coma.

EYES OPEN:	
Spontaneously	4
To speech	3
To pain	2
Never	1
BEST MOTOR RESPONSE:	
Obeys commands	6
Localises pain	5
Flexion withdrawal	4
Decorticate flexion	3
Decerebrate extension	2
No response	1
BEST VERBAL RESPONSE:	
Orientated	5
Confused	4
Inappropriate words	3
Incomprehensible sounds	2
Silent	1

REVISED TRAUMA SCORE
Provides a general assessment of physiological derangement.

	CODED VALUE	X WEIGHT= SCORE
RESPIRATORY RATE		
10-29	4	
>29	3	0.2908
6-9	2	
1-5	1	
0	0	
SYSTOLIC BLOOD PRESSURE		
>89	4	
76-89	3	0.7326
50-75	2	
1-49	1	
0	0	
GLASGOW COMA SCALE		
13-15	4	
9-12	3	0.9368
6-8	2	
4-5	1	
3	0	

Example: a man falls from a ladder and is admitted with a Glasgow coma score calculated as follows: eyes open to pain (2), localising pain (5), and using inappropriate words (3). This gives a total of 10. He is tachypnoeic with a respiratory rate of 35/min and his systolic blood pressure is 80 mmHg. His RTS is as follows:

Respiratory rate score	3 x 0.2908 =	0.8724
Systolic score	3 x 0.7326 =	2.1978
GCS score	3 x 0.9368 =	2.8104
Total RTS	=	5.8806

The highest, and most favourable, score is 7.8408; the worst is 0.

APACHE II SCORE

This provides an indicator of performance; it does not predict outcome, although the sickest patients have the highest scores. It is usually calculated by a computer programme, which will ask for parameters to be entered at a keyboard; it is thus not necessary to know the score attached to a particular parameter, although it is useful to have an overview of how the score is calculated.

A. ACUTE PHYSIOLOGY SCORE
Score 0 (normal) to +4 (high or low abnormal)

TEMPERATURE
MEAN ARTERIAL PRESSURE
HEART RATE
RESPIRATORY RATE
A-aDO$_2$
ARTERIAL pH
SERUM SODIUM
SERUM POTASSIUM
SERUM CREATININE
HAEMATOCRIT
LEUCOCYTES
GLASGOW COMA SCORE

B. AGE POINTS

Age:	<44	45-54	55-64	65-74	>75
Points:	0	2	3	5	7

C. CHRONIC HEALTH POINTS
Elective postoperative admission: 2 points
Emergency, chronic liver disease, CVS, RS, Renal disease or immunocompromise: 5 points.

GOLDMAN CARDIAC RISK INDEX

FACTOR	POINTS
Third heart sound or elevated JVP	11
MI within 6 months	10
Rhythm other than sinus rhythm	7
Ventricular ectopics more than 5/min	7
Age over 70	5
Emergency operation	4
Tight aortic stenosis	3
Poor general condition	3
Thoracic/abdominal operation	3

Risk of cardiac death with a score over 25 is 56%. Note that Goldman did not include angina or hypertension; this has been disputed by other authorities.

LUNN & MUSHIN 1982: INCIDENCE OF CVS DISEASE
This is useful data to have in mind when dealing with anaesthesia in the elderly; however well the patient may seem, cardiovascular disease will be present in a large number even though it may be covert.

Age 40-50 = 6%
Age 50-60 = 23%
Age 60-70 = 45%
Age >70 = 100%

REINFARCTION FROM ANAESTHESIA
This occurs on 3rd postoperative day and has 50-70% mortality.

MONTHS since infarct	STEEN, 1978	RAO, 1983
0-3	35%	5%
3-6	12%	3%
>6	5%	1%

Rao described aggressive, invasive pre- and postoperative therapy, producing greater safety for the patient with the recent myocardial infarction presenting for surgery.

Never been reproduced!

MILLER DYSPNOEA GRADES
This provides a useful means of quantifying cardiopulmonary function.
0 : No breathlessness
1 : Can walk any distance, but needs time;
2 : Breathless at 100 metres;
3 : Can walk a few yards only;
4 : Breathless at rest.

THE ELECTROCARDIOGRAM

This is a brief aid to analysing the electrocardiogram in a methodical
fashion.
1. NAME and AGE; make sure the ECG belongs to the correct patient
2. GAIN: 10 mm/mV
3. RECORDING RATE: 25 mm/sec is usual, but 50 mm/sec may be used
to analyse a tachycardia
4. RHYTHM
5. HEART RATE: small square (ssq) = 0.04 sec, large square =
0.2 sec: heart rate = 300/n of large squares between complexes
6. AXIS: using I and aVf as vectors
7. P WAVES should be < 3 ssq. wide, < 2.5 high in II
8. PR INTERVAL should be 0.12 - 0.2 sec, 3 - 5 ssq.
9. QRS: Duration should be < 3 ssq; look for Q waves, R progression and
R & S amplitude.
10. ST SEGMENTS
11. QT INTERVAL; QT corrected (QTc) = QT/ $\sqrt{RR}$ interval (normal
QTc <0.44 sec)
12. T WAVES ? U WAVES

New York Heart Association

I - no funct. limit
II - slight funct limit
III - Marked funct limit.
    no symptoms at rest
IV - unable to perform any
    activity

19

DISEASE PATTERNS ON ECG

1. HYPERTROPHIC CONDITIONS

- LEFT VENTRICULAR HYPERTROPHY (LVH): Left axis deviation (LAD), tall R in V5,6, deep S in V2; T inversion in I, II, III, V5,6
- RIGHT VENTRICULAR HYPERTROPHY (RVH): Right axis deviation (RAD), tall R in V1-4, R=S in V5; T inversion V1,2.
- LEFT ATRIAL HYPERTROPHY (LAH): Broad notched P.
- RIGHT ATRIAL HYPERTROPHY (RAH): Tall peaked P.

2. DEFECTS OF RHYTHM

- ATRIAL FIBRILLATION (AF): No P waves, QRS irregularly irregular.
- ATRIAL FLUTTER: P rate 300/min, variable conduction.
- ATRIAL EXTRASYSTOLE: Abnormal P, normal QRS.
- NODAL EXTRASYSTOLE: No P, normal QRS.
- VENTRICULAR EXTRASYSTOLE: No P, abnormal QRS.
- BIGEMINY: Ventricular ectopic (VE) coupled to a normal PQRST.
- ESCAPE: Nodal ectopic or VE during sinus arrest or bradycardia.
- SINUS TACHYCARDIA: Rate <150/min.
- SUPRAVENTRICULAR TACHYCARDIA: Rate usually >150/min, no P waves; often nodal in origin.
- BROAD COMPLEX TACHYCARDIA: usually ventricular in origin (suggested by deep S in V6) or junctional with a bundle branch block (dominant R in V1).
- VENTRICULAR TACHYCARDIA (VT): Defined as >3 VE in a salvo.
- VF: Chaos.
- TORSADE DES POINTES: VT of writhing morphology.

Inotropy — ↑ force of contraction

Chronotropy — ↑ freq of impulse from pacema...

Dromotropy — ↑ speed of conduction

Bathmotropy — ↑ excitability by altering threshold potential.

3. DEFECTS OF CONDUCTION

- WOLFF-PARKINSON-WHITE (WPW): short PR, δ-wave before QRS.
- FIRST DEGREE ATRIO-VENTRICULAR (AV) BLOCK: >0.2 sec (5 ssq).
- SECOND DEGREE A-V BLOCK (MOBITZ 2): Most beats normally conducted, occasional P not followed by QRS.
- WENCKEBACH A-V BLOCK: Progressive prolongation of PR until non-conduction occurs.
- THIRD DEGREE (COMPLETE) A-V BLOCK: Dissociation of P from QRS.
- RIGHT BUNDLE BRANCH BLOCK (RBBB): QRS > 0.12 sec (3 ssq), RAD, MaRRoW (QRS morphology changes from M shape to W shape across anterior chest leads).
- LEFT BUNDLE BRANCH BLOCK(LBBB): QRS > 0.12 sec (3 ssq), WiLLiaM (QRS morphology opposite to RBBB), T inversion.
- LEFT ANTERIOR HEMIBLOCK: QRS > 0.12 sec (3 ssq), LAD.

4. CORONARY VASCULAR DISORDERS

- MYOCARDIAL INFARCTION (MI): ST elevation, Q waves, T inversion in affected leads.
- ISCHAEMIA: ST depression horizontally, commonly in lateral leads.
- PERICARDITIS: ST depression concave upwards, all leads.
- PULMONARY EMBOLISM (PE): S>R in I, Q in III, T inversion in III; RAD.

5. ELECTROLYTES AND DRUGS

- HYPOKALAEMIA: Long QT, flat T, U wave.
- HYPERKALAEMIA: Tall peaked T.
- HYPOCALCAEMIA: Long QT.
- DIGITALIS: ST down slope, T inversion.

THE CHEST X-RAY

1. NAME, LABELLED SIDE; the name may reveal that the patient is at particular risk of, for example, pulmonary tuberculosis; the age is relevant in interpretation of pathological changes.

2. P-A or A-P; the latter are often portable films, taken in Accident and Emergency or Intensive Care, and evaluation of the heart size may be inappropriate.

3. HARDWARE; endotracheal tube, central venous cannulae, drains.

4. ROTATION; from position of clavicles in relation to vertebral column.

5. PENETRATION; it should be able to define thoracic vertebrae with correct penetration.

6. SOFT TISSUES; breasts, surgical emphysema.

7. BONY SKELETON; ribs, spine; metastatic diseases, fractures

8. TRACHEA; size, deviation in malignant disease or pneumothorax

9. UPPER MEDIASTINUM; loss of definition indicates collapse of adjacent lobe. Increased diameter suggests vascular trauma.

10. LUNG FIELDS; pneumothorax, fluid, vessels; increased density with loss of volume is collapse, increased density without loss of volume implies consolidation.

11. HILA; position, fissures.

12. DIAPHRAGM: costo-phrenic angles, for effusions, gas beneath in perforated viscus.

13. HEART AND AORTA: loss of definition indicates collapse of adjacent lobe

14. HIDDEN AREAS: behind diaphragm and heart, apices.

ARTERIAL BLOOD GASES

When examining a blood gas result, it is wise to be methodical.
1. $PaCO_2$ is related to ventilatory status
2. Consider pH in context of $PaCO_2$ (see below)
3. PaO_2 with inspired O_2 fraction implies hypoxic status

$$pH \propto \frac{HCO_3}{CO_2}$$

Only a certain number of combinations exist, and diagnosis can be based on three patterns of ventilation; low, normal or high $PaCO_2$.

ALVEOLAR HYPERVENTILATION : $PaCO2 < 3.8$ kPa
a. pH > 7.5	= acute hyperventilation
b. pH 7.4 - 7.5	= chronic hyperventilation
c. pH 7.3 - 7.4	= partly compensated metabolic acidosis
d. pH < 7.3	= metabolic acidosis

NORMAL VENTILATION : $PaCO2$ 3.8 - 6.8 kPa
a. pH > 7.5	= acute metabolic alkalosis
b. pH < 7.3	= acute metabolic acidosis

RESPIRATORY FAILURE : $PaCO2 > 6.8$ kPa
a. pH > 7.5	= partly compensated metabolic alkalosis
b. pH 7.3 - 7.5	= chronic ventilatory failure
c. pH < 7.3	= acute ventilatory failure

NUNN 1988 NORTHWICK PARK

This was a paper describing 42 cases of severe respiratory disease presenting for surgery, all having general anaesthesia. They all had FEV1 less than 1.0 litre. Only 4 of the 42 required postoperative ventilation. The conclusion is that best predictors of requirement for postoperative ventilation are:

1. $PaO2 < 7.2$ kPa
2. Dyspnoea at rest

(*Anaesthesia* 1988: **43**, 543-51)

SIMPLIFIED DAVENPORT DIAGRAM

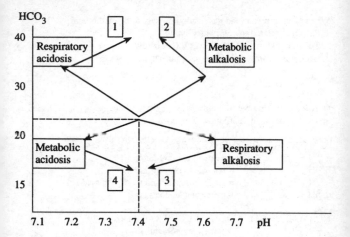

Compensation occurs towards the 7.4 line, i.e. renal H⁺ excretion and HCO₃ retention as shown.

1 = Renal (Metabolic) compensation for respiratory acidosis
2 = Respiratory compensation for metabolic alkalosis
3 = Renal (metabolic) compensation for respiratory alkalosis
4 = Respiratory compensation for metabolic acidosis

Respiratory correction depends on increasing or decreasing minute volume and happens rapidly, over the course of a few minutes. Renal correction depends on bicarbonate retention by the kidney and is a chronic phenomenon, taking hours to days to happen.

DAY SURGERY UNIT SELECTION CRITERIA

Day surgery may account for more than 50% of elective general surgery. There are financial, patient-satisfaction and waiting list imperatives driving the development of day surgery.

THESE EXAMPLES ARE APPROPRIATE FOR DAY SURGERY:
General surgery; hernia repair, varicose veins, circumcision, removal skin lesions, sigmoidoscopy, lymph node biopsy.
Urology; cystoscopy, vasectomy, excision epididymal cyst.
Gynaecology; dilatation and curettage, laparoscopy (including sterilisation), termination of pregnancy.
Orthopaedics; arthroscopy, change of plaster, release trigger finger.
Dental; conservation, extractions, frenectomy, removal of metal.
Ear, nose and throat: myringotomy, polypectomy, examination under anaesthesia.

THE FOLLOWING ARE INCONSISTENT WITH DAY SURGERY:
Medical; ischaemic heart disease, advanced hypertension, congestive cardiac failure, bleeding disorders, diabetes mellitus, obesity with body mass index over 33, muscular disease, poorly controlled epilepsy.
Surgical and anaesthetic; malignant hyperpyrexia susceptibility, previous anaphylactic reaction to anaesthesia. Scoline apnoea is controversial.
Social; no transport, telephone or supervision for 24 hours.

ABDOMINAL AORTIC ANEURISM: SELECTION FOR SURGERY

HISTORY: with special reference to other symptoms of cardiovascular disease:
- Amaurosis fugax
- Ischaemic chest pain
- Exercise tolerance
- Orthopnoea
- Mesenteric angina
- Claudication

EXAMINATION: peripheral pulses, heart rhythm, rate and sounds

INVESTIGATIONS: In the first instance,
- ECG
- Chest XRay

Evaluate Goldman Cardiac Risk Index

```
No major risk factor  ←→  Risk factors identified
       ↓                          ↓
   CLASS I              Dipyridamole-Thallium scan*
                          ↙               ↘
              No reversible defect    Reversible defect
                      ↓                      ↓
                  CLASS II              Angiography
                                        ↙        ↘
                                  CLASS III    Class IV
   ┌─────────┐                       ↓            ↓
   │ SURGERY │ ←───────        Myocardial      Serial
   └─────────┘              revascularisation  assessment,
                                              conservative
                                              management
```

*This uses injected thallium-201 which is taken up into cardiac muscle in proportion to the degree of perfusion. The isotope is detected with a gamma-camera, demonstrating hypo-perfused areas, which can be scarred or ischaemic. The distinction is made by injecting a coronary vasodilator, such as dipyridamole; if an area is reversibly ischaemic, it will dilate and light up after administration of dipyridamole. It may then be appropriate to revascularise such areas before elective surgery.

HAEMOGLOBINOPATHIES

These are disorders of haemoglobin synthesis. The important distinction is between Sickle cell disease, which is a qualitative defect, and Thalassaemia, which is a group of quantitative disorders.

SICKLE CELL DISEASE
Sickle cell disease is acquired by autosomal dominant inheritance, and is found in the Afro-Caribbean and Mediterranean populations. The β-chain of HbA has valine substituted for glutamine at position 6. Heterozygotes are at risk of pulmonary infarcts but protected against malaria. Symptoms in homozygotes occur as acute pain in chest, bone (especially of the femoral head), abdomen, and over the spleen; there may also be cerebrovascular accident or myocardial infarction.
PRECIPITANTS include: hypoxia, acidosis, dehydration, hypothermia, and the use of tourniquets. Homozygotes rarely survive beyond age 50.
DIAGNOSIS: Sickledex test: the reagent is Na metabisulphite. Electrophoresis is then required to distinguish sickle cell trait from sickle cell disease. Exchange transfusion is indicated if HbA is less 40% of haemoglobin, or if total Hb < 10 g/dl.

THALASSAEMIA
This results in a partial (heterozygous, thalassaemia minor) or a complete (homozygous, thalassaemia major) abnormality in the α-chain or β-chain of haemoglobin. α-thalassaemia, because the α-chain is universal to all Hb, is fatal in the major form. β-thalassaemia is the commonest.

As well as these two, there are as many as 100 other haemoglobinopathies which may exist alone or in combination with the above. The commonest of these is HbSC.

PAEDIATRIC ILLNESSES

These notes are intended to jog the memory when called to see a condition which you may not have seen in your recent practice.

PYLORIC STENOSIS

The incidence is 1:350, of whom 85% are male. There is a $\downarrow K^+, \downarrow Cl^-$ alkalosis with paradoxical urinary excretion of H^+ to maintain Na^+; resuscitation takes priority over surgery.

Fluid required for correction (ml) = 2/3 body weight x (106 - [Cl])

Methods:

1. Rapid sequence induction.
2. Gas induction
3. Awake intubation
4. Local

TRACHEOESOPHAGEAL FISTULA

The incidence is 1:3500, males affected equally with females. 85% have a blind oesophageal pouch with fistula distal to trachea. An awake intubation is usual, situating a plain oral tracheal tube distal to the fistula.

CONGENITAL DIAPHRAGMATIC HERNIA

The incidence is 1:5000, females are twice as commonly affected as males. 80% are left sided (Foramen of Bochdalek). 20% also have a cardiovascular defect. Only 50% survive, those with accompanying pulmonary dysplasia doing worse.

OMPHALOCOELE: The incidence is 1:5000. It is a persistence of the herniation of the gut into the extra-embryonic part of the umbilical cord. The gut is covered by a membrane. Other defects are associated.

GASTROSCHISIS: The incidence of this condition is 1:30000. This is an ischaemic defect of the anterior abdominal wall, with prolapse of the gut through the defect; the gut is not covered. There are no associations.

CONGENITAL HEART DEFECTS: These are generally seen in females more than in males, and can be divided into those lesions associated with cyanosis and those not.

ACYANOTIC	CYANOTIC
Ventricular septal defect (VSD) Atrial septal defect (ASD) Patent ductus arteriosus (PDA) Pulmonary stenosis Aortic stenosis Coarctation of the aorta Hypoplastic heart	Transposition of the great vessels Tetralogy of Fallot Eisenmengers (a late consequence of prolonged left to right shunt with eventual reversal of pressures)

"Left to right, pink and mighty; right to left, blue and unsightly"
If a shunt goes left to right, effort is wasted and hypertrophy occurs; if a shunt goes right to left, deoxygenated blood is pumped into the systemic circulation and cyanosis occurs.

VSD:
This is the commonest congenital cardiovascular lesion seen in neonates. It is characterised by a pan-systolic murmur at the left sternal edge and biventricular hypertrophy.
ASD:
This may present in the adult; features are an ejection systolic murmur in the pulmonary area, a fixed split second heart sound, and right ventricular hypertrophy.
PDA:
There is a continuous murmur in the pulmonary area, and left ventricular hypertrophy.
COARCTATION:
The classic sign is a pan systolic murmur, radiating to the back. Chest Xray may show rib notching due to engorged collateral circulation. There will be left ventricular hypertrophy.

CYSTIC FIBROSIS: The incidence is 1:2000 many of whom now reach adulthood. The inheritance is autosomal recessive, with 1:25 carrying the gene, which is on chromosome 7, where more than 200 mutations have been recorded. The underlying defect is of abnormal epithelial Cl^- and Na^+ transport resulting in increased electrolyte content of secretions. Presentation is by meconium ileus or, in later childhood, recurrent chest infections (chest illness or heart disease are the cause of death in 95% of affected adults) or malabsorption. Diagnosis is by pilocarpine iontophoresis.

Indications for surgery include bowel surgery in the neonate, polypectomy or vascular access in childhood, and transplantation in the adult. Active chest infection should be excluded before elective surgery. Electrolyte disturbance (hypokalaemia and hypochloraemia) should be corrected. Desaturation occurs readily and securing the airway by intubation and ventilation is usual. A volatile is useful for bronchodilation. Regional anaesthesia is helpful in the postoperative period for aiding physiotherapy.

CONNECTIVE TISSUE DISEASES

Although these conditions are common and of considerable clinical significance to the anaesthetist, they are over-represented in examinations.

CONSIDER: Under each condition, think about the patient, and the anaesthetic.
- Patient: condition and operation type which may be associated with the condition, for example, arthroplasty in rheumatoid arthritis.
- Systems: Effects of the condition on the cardiovascular, respiratory, musculoskeletal, renal, and central nervous systems. Remember the use of drugs.
- Anaesthesia: Operation, premedication, induction, airway control, postoperative management. Cervical collars. Deep vein thrombosis and pulmonary embolus prophylaxis.

DIAGNOSIS OF CONNECTIVE TISSUE DISEASE:
Erythrocyte sedimentation rate (ESR); rheumatoid factor; antinuclear factor; biopsies of muscle, temporal artery, and kidney.

RHEUMATOID:
Seen from age 30, eventually affecting 1% population, 3:1 female to male. There is a 10% association with pericarditis. Anaemia of chronic disease is almost universal. 2% will have fibrosing alveolitis and ↓ compliance. Peptic ulceration is common. 25% will have occipito-atlanto-axial joint

XRay changes, but only 6% will have symptoms. Anticipate a difficult view of the airway; 53% in one series were Cormack and Lehane grade 3 or 4. The use of steroids is common.

SCLERODERMA:
This is a disease of the middle-aged. It is associated with pulmonary fibrosis, achalasia, polymyositis, and renal failure. The multisystem manifestations of the disease therefore present considerable challenges to the anaesthetist.

SYSTEMIC LUPUS ERYTHEMATOSUS:
The incidence is 1:10000, with a sex difference of 8:1 female to male. There may be pericarditis, mitral endocarditis (Libman-Sacks), pulmonary fibrosis, and nephrotic syndrome. The use of steroids is common.

POLYARTERITIS NODOSA: Males and females are equally affected. The features are hypertension, asthma, nephrotic syndrome, infarcts and cerebrovascular accidents. Steroids are usually prescribed.

NEUROLOGICAL DISEASES

EPILEPSY: Avoid methohexitone and enflurane, both of which are epileptogenic.

BELL'S PALSY: This is a lower motor neurone lesion and affects the upper part of the face as well as the lower part, in contrast to an upper motor neurone lesion, which will spare the upper part.

HORNER'S SYNDROME: This is a sympathetic lesion; everything gets smaller or contracts; the features are therefore a small pupil (miosis), enophthalmos, anhidrosis, ptosis, stuffy nose and flushed skin. It may be associated with a high regional block or with malignant disease (Pancoast tumour of the apex of the lung).

III NERVE PALSY: This produces ptosis with an enlarged pupil (mydriasis).

TENTORIAL CONING: This produces 3rd cranial nerve palsy, ↓HR, ↑BP, ↓GCS.

MEDULLARY CONING: Associated with ↓respiratory rate and neck stiffness.

HYDROCEPHALUS: Cerebrospinal fluid (CSF) production is 0.3 ml/min in adult, from choroid plexus in the lateral and 3rd ventricles. The total volume is 120 ml and turnover takes place every 4-6 hours. CSF is absorbed from arachnoid villi in proportion to the difference between CSF pressure and central venous pressure. In children, it may be associated with spina bifida, from a congenital aquaduct stenosis, or as a result of intracranial bleeding or infection.

BULBAR PALSIES: The significance of these is that they represent a hazard to airway safety; they fall into two groups:

	Pseudobulbar palsy	**Bulbar palsy**
Cause	Cerebrovascular accident, multiple sclerosis	Motor neurone disease, Guillain-Barré syndrome
Feature	UPPER motor neurone lesion	LOWER motor neurone lesion
Emotion	Labile	Normal
Tongue	Spastic	Fasciculating
Jaw jerk	Increased	Absent

MUSCULAR DISEASES

MULTIPLE SCLEROSIS (MS): The incidence is 50/100,000. An environmental cause is suspected from the geographical variation in the condition. Diagnosis is made by magnetic resonance imaging. Of those that present with optic neuritis, 50% progress to MS. Symptoms worsen with stress and heat. Suxamethonium causes K^+ release. Regional techniques are acceptable, but carry a theoretical risk of accelerating demyelination.

MUSCULAR DYSTROPHIES: Cardiac muscle is involved. Suxamethonium causes extreme K^+ release. Patients are sensitive to non-depolarising neuromuscular blockers.

MYOTONIA DYSTROPHICA: This is a disease transmitted by autosomal dominant inheritance. The features are of wasting, balding, cataracts, diabetes mellitus, and intraventricular conduction defects. Suxamethonium causes excessive K^+ release, and intense myotonia (which can also be caused by neostigmine). Local anaesthetics and regional blocks cause prolonged weakness, including uterine atony. The safe anaesthetic includes propofol, non-depolarising muscle blockers, and opiates. Neostigmine is not safe.

GUILLAIN-BARRÉ: This is an acute postinfective polyneuropathy; it occurs 7-10 days after an infectious (usually viral) illness, producing an ascending paralysis. Maximum disability occurs at 4 weeks.

MYASTHENIA GRAVIS: This is characterised by antibodies to postsynaptic acetylcholine receptors, causing weakness of neuromuscular transmission. It is associated with thymoma. Edrophonium reverses weakness for 10 minutes and is the basis of the diagnostic "Tensilon test".

EATON-LAMBERT SYNDROME: A disorder of acetylcholine release, in contrast to myasthenia gravis, which affects the receptor. It is associated with oat cell carcinoma. Muscle function improves with movement, and the Tensilon test is negative, distinguishing it from myasthenia.

DISORDERS OF CONSCIOUSNESS

Consciousness has content and level, and conscious behaviour requires:
>   1. Intact cerebral cortex.
>   2. Ascending reticular activating system.
>   3. Input of sensory or thought processes.

COMA: "Not obeying any commands, not uttering any words, not opening the eyes".

LOCKED-IN SYNDROME: This is a disorder of the content of consciousness. Causes are pontine or midbrain CVA, or tumour. 60% will not survive.

PERSISTENT VEGETATIVE STATE: This is a disorder of the state of consciousness. There is a functional brain stem, with a damaged cortex (reduced blood flow, retarded visual evoked responses). 45% are due to head injury, 40% to CVA.

BRAIN STEM DEATH: This is described as having 2 preconditions, 6 exclusions, and 7 criteria. See below.

PORPHYRIA

There are broadly two groups of porphyria; erythropoetic and hepatic. Anaesthetic drugs do not precipitate erythropoetic forms. The basis of the condition is induction of the small, inducible enzyme δaminolaevulinic acid synthetase by pregnancy, diet, infection, alcohol, and drugs including steroids and barbiturates. There is then a deficient enzyme further down the synthetic pathway of haem; small intermediates cross the blood-brain barrier, causing psychological manifestations; larger ones do not, and cause cutaneous manifestations instead.

ACUTE INTERMITTENT PORPHYRIA: Seen in Scandanavia, causing psychosis, defect is protoporphyrinogen I synthase. Diagnosis is based on finding ALA in urine.

VARIEGATE PORPHYRIA: Seen in South Africa, affecting skin, defect is protoporphyrinogen oxidase. Diagnosis from finding porphyrins in stool.

The safe anaesthetic includes propofol, nitrous (but probably not other volatiles), vecuronium, opiates, and domperidone. Local anaesthetics are contentious.

LIVER DISEASE

TESTS:
EXCRETORY FUNCTION: Bilirubin. If unconjugated, this implies excessive haemolysis or hepatic failure, and the bilirubin will be lipid soluble and enters central nervous system. Only conjugated, water soluble, bilirubin, may appear in urine and the presence of this indicates biliary obstruction.
CELL DAMAGE: Indicated by elevated transaminases. Hepatitis causes increase in ALT over AST; tumour and sepsis cause increase in AST more than ALT. Alcohol characteristically causes elevated γGT.
CHOLESTASIS: This is indicated by elevated alkaline phosphatase.
SYNTHETIC FUNCTION: This is related to albumin level, and a defect of synthetic function will prolong the prothrombin time.
SCORING IN LIVER DISEASE:
CHILD: Class A-B-C; based on bilirubin, albumin level, presence of ascites, whether there is a neurological disorder, and the nutritional status.
PUGH: Score 4 -12; based on bilirubin levels, albumin, prothrombin time, and whether there is encephalopathy. A score less than 6 implies good risk, but over10 indicates a poor operative risk.
SAFE ANAESTHETIC IN LIVER DISEASE: Includes fluid rehydration, avoidance of hypotension and care with regionals in case of impaired clotting. Thiopentone, atracurium and isoflurane are acceptable. The risk is of further liver impairment and of the hepatorenal syndrome.

RENAL DISEASE

TESTS:
FOR RENAL PLASMA FLOW: PAH clearance. Normal = 625 ml/min.
FOR GLOMERULAR FILTRATION RATE: Creatinine clearance.
Normal = 125 ml/min. EDTA clearance confirms normal function (prior to transplant) but does not quantify abnormality.
FILTRATION FRACTION = Glomerular filtration rate/Renal plasma flow.

Kidney disease can present in only four ways:
        1. Proteinuria; if extreme, this is the nephrotic syndrome.
        2. Haematuria.
        3. Uraemia; acute or chronic, with consequences, e.g. hypertension.
        4. Hypertension

PROTEINURIA: Exists if elimination of protein in urine exceeds 150 mg/24h; if more than 5 g/24h and hypoalbuminaemia is present, this is the nephrotic syndrome.
Causes of proteinuria:

1. Pyelonephritis (acute and chronic).
2. Glomerulonephritis (acute and chronic).
3. Obstructive nephropathy.
4. Congestive cardiac failure.
5. Postural.
6. Diabetes mellitus.
7. Myeloma.
8. Nephrotic syndrome, which in turn may be due to:

a. Minimal change glomerulonephritis (80%)
b. Diabetes mellitus.
c. Systemic lupus erythematosus.
d. Heavy metal poisoning (Fanconi's syndrome).

HAEMATURIA: Exists if, in the urine, there is elimination of:
Erythrocytes: 1×10^6 cells/24h (2 per High power field, HPF), or
Leucocytes: 2×10^6 cells/24h (4 per HPF)
Causes of haematuria:

1. Calculi.
2. Tumours: bladder, kidneys, prostate.
3. Urinary tract infection.
4. Trauma.
5. Acute glomerulonephritis: Acute streptococcal glomerulonephritis causes the nephritic syndrome of haematuria and oliguria proceeding to oedema.
6. Malignant hypertension.
7. Benign prostatic hypertrophy.
8. Connective tissue disease: Systemic lupus erythematosus (SLE), polyarteritis nodosa (PAN).
9. Infective endocarditis.
10. Anticoagulants.

ACUTE RENAL FAILURE: This is present when urine output is less than 400 ml/24h.
Causes of renal failure:

1. Pre-renal; hypovolaemia, shock.
2. Post-renal; obstruction.
3. Renal parenchymal:

a. glomerulonephritis.
b. Pregnancy induced hypertension.

c. Acute tubular necrosis; a dilute oliguria occurs with high filling pressures: It is often a consequence of acute renal failure, and is often self limiting after up to 3 weeks of fluid restriction or dialysis. Recovery is heralded by a diuresis and natriuresis.

d. Malignant hypertension

e. Connective tissue disease.

f. Septicaemia.

g. Disseminated intravascular coagulation.

h Hepatorenal syndrome.

SAFE ANAESTHETIC IN RENAL DISEASE: Includes thiopentone, atracurium, non-depolarising blockade (suxamethonium may have unpredictable duration of action, although many would advocate a rapid sequence induction), and a volatile. Meticulous attention to renal output is required.

Dose in renal failure = Usual dose x $\dfrac{\text{normal t½}}{\text{observed t½}}$

PLASMA CHOLINESTERASE GENOTYPES

An abnormal response to suxamethonium, if due to an abnormal form of plasma cholinesterase, may result in prolongation of action, sometimes for several hours. The management involves maintenance of the airway, supporting ventilation, and sedation until the block wears off. The patient, and first-degree relatives, must then be investigated.

Geno-type	Incidence	Response to suxamethonium	DN	FN
EuEu	96%	Normal	80	60
EaEa	1:2800	Very prolonged	20	20
EuEa	1:25	Slightly prolonged	40-60	45
EfEf	1:154000	Mod. prolonged	70	30
EsEs	1:100000	Very prolonged		
EuEf	1:200	Slightly prolonged	75	50
EuEs	1:190	Slightly prolonged	80	60
EaEf	1:20000	Mod. prolonged	45	35
EsEa	1:29000	Very prolonged	20	19
EfEs	1:150000	Mod. prolonged	60	35

DN= dibucaine number; FN= fluoride number. The dibucaine number is the % inhibition of enzyme by dibucaine, 10^{-5} M concentration. Normal inhibition is 80%. A homozygous defect results in an abnormal enzyme with reduced affinity for suxamethonium. This also happens to be resistant to dibucaine inhibition. Fluoride inhibition may also be used to further identify the particular genotype; because there are 4 alleles, there are 10 possible genotypes.

PSYCHIATRIC DRUGS

MONOAMINE OXIDASE INHIBITORS: (MAOI)
Direct-acting agents (adrenaline, noradrenaline) have no enhanced effect in the presence of MAOI, since adrenaline and noradrenaline both act post-synaptically, whereas MAOI block intraneuronal breakdown. Indirect acting agents (ephedrine), however, are taken up and displace neurotransmitter and in combination with MAOI can precipitate hypertension and subarachnoid haemorrhage, as can pethidine.

TRICYCLIC ANTIDEPRESSANTS:
These act by blockade of reuptake, and could present a risk of enhanced effect in the presence of direct-acting vasopressors. Their phenothiazine nucleus also confers an antimuscarinic effect. They are arrhythmogenic, especially in the elderly.

SELECTIVE SEROTONIN UPTAKE INHIBITORS:
Experience of these (fluoxetine, Prozac) is limited, but co-administration
with MAOI can precipitate a neuroleptic-malignant syndrome like event
for which dantrolene may be of use.

LITHIUM: This enhances the effect of neuromuscular blockers, and
induction agents. It also carries a risk of renal damage in hypovolaemia.

STEROIDS

ADRENOCORTICAL INSUFFICIENCY: This occurs in sepsis,
tuberculous adrenalitis (Addison's disease), and the Waterhouse-
Friderichsen syndrome (haemorrhage into adrenals). The main concern
however is from steroid therapy, whether oral, topical, inhaled or
parenteral, which will suppress the pituitary-adrenal axis. Beware also the
depot steroids used for chronic pain and atopy. Endogenous cortisol output
is 25 mg/day rising to 500 mg/day in stress, which response may not be
possible if adrenal suppression exists. This may precipitate an Addisonian
crisis, which consists of collapse, hyperkalaemia, hyponatraemia, and
hypoglycaemia.

EQUIVALENCE:
>Hydrocortisone 100 mg
>Prednisolone   25 mg
>Betamethasone 4 mg
>Dexamethasone 4 mg

REPLACEMENT: Hydrocortisone 100 mg at induction then reduce from
100 mg qds over three days.

BLOOD PRODUCTS

All donated blood starts as 450 ml from the donor, with 60 ml additive, cooled to 4°c.

CAPD = citrate, adenine, phosphate, dextrose
SAGM = sodium chloride, adenine, glucose, mannitol

Random blood	64%	compatible
ABO cross-match	99.4%	compatible
ABO + Rh cross-match	99.8%	compatible
Full cross-match	99.95%	compatible

Product	Vol. (ml)	Additive	Hct	Life
Whole blood	450	60 ml CAPD	0.45	21days
Plasma-reduced	350	60 ml CAPD	0.60	21days
SAGM	280	100 ml SAGM	0.60	45days
Conc. red cells	200	minimum	0.80	
Human Albumin	450	pasteurised 60°C		
FFP(all factors)	200	stored at -30°C		6months
Cryoppt(f8 esp)	15	stored at -30°C		6months
Platelets	6units increase platelet count by 30,000/dl			3 days

Stored blood has the following characteristics: pH 6.9, K^+ 20 mmol/l, HCO_3 10 mmol/l.

Filters: A100 = 180 μm; depth or screen = 20-40 μm. When transfusing platelets, use either special platelet filter, or none at all; ordinary filters will block.

CARDIAC VALVES

FOR ALL CASES:
Tests will include an electrocardiogram (ECG), chest XRay (CXR), and full blood count (FBC). An echocardiogram may be helpful to assess the appearance of a valve, the pressure gradient across it, the ejection fraction, and ventricular wall motion and thickening. If on therapy, urea and electrolytes (U&E) are indicated. If cardiovascularly compromised, a pulmonary artery catheter is necessary. A medical opinion may be valuable in order to optimise therapy. Remember endocarditis prophylaxis.

Avoid regional techniques, especially with stenotic lesions. The sympathetic block induced in the presence of a fixed output state will cause a catastrophic fall in blood pressure.

AORTIC STENOSIS:
Causes: Calcified bicuspid valve or rheumatic heart disease.
Important signs: Ejection systolic murmur, low pulse pressure, chest pain, left ventricular failure, syncope. Sudden death is a feature of this condition.
Key:
- Provide adequate filling pressure.
- Maintain systemic vascular resistance (SVR).
- Control heart rate.

MITRAL STENOSIS:
Causes: Rheumatic heart disease.
Important signs: Mid diastolic murmur, atrial fibrillation (AF), emboli, haemoptysis, right ventricular failure.
Points: Often anticoagulated; may be hypovolaemic from diuretic tharapy. An ECG is mandatory to establish rhythm.
Key:
- Control ventricular rate and maintain sinus rhythm.
- Adequate filling pressure.
- Maintain systemic vascular resistance.
- Avoid pulmonary vasoconstriction.

MANAGEMENT OF PAEDIATRIC MURMURS

This is a common problem; what to do when confronted by a murmur in a child scheduled for surgery, when there will probably not be time to organise preoperative investigation.

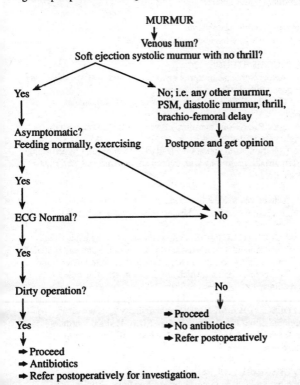

MURMUR

↓

Venous hum?

Soft ejection systolic murmur with no thrill?

Yes

↓

No; i.e. any other murmur, PSM, diastolic murmur, thrill, brachio-femoral delay

↓

Asymptomatic?
Feeding normally, exercising

↓

Postpone and get opinion

Yes

↓

ECG Normal? ⟶ No

Yes

↓

Dirty operation?

No

↓

→ Proceed
→ No antibiotics
→ Refer postoperatively

Yes

↓

→ Proceed
→ Antibiotics
→ Refer postoperatively for investigation.

AORTIC INCOMPETENCE:
Causes: Acute: Subacute bacterial endocarditis (SBE), Marfan's;
requires emergency aortic valve replacement.
              Chronic: Rheumatic heart disease
Important signs: Early diastolic murmur, waterhammer pulse, left
ventricular dilation and failure.
Key:
- Slight tachycardia is beneficial
- Avoid increasing systemic vascular resistance.

MITRAL INCOMPETENCE:
Causes: Acute: Subacute bacterial endocarditis and post MI; these may
need emergency mitral valve replacement
              Chronic: Rheumatic heart disease and left ventricular
hypertrophy.
Important signs: Pansystolic murmur, left ventricular failure, with or
without right ventricular failure.
Points: Left ventricular dilatation may lead to left ventricular hypertrophy
and so to left atrial hypertrophy with pulmonary oedema and then right
ventricular failure.
Key:
- Slight tachycardia may be beneficial.
- Avoid increasing systemic and pulmonary vascular resistance.

OTHER VALVULAR LESIONS: Pulmonary stenosis, which is usually
congenital, and tricuspid incompetence which is seen in subacute bacterial
endocarditis and in drug addicts; an important feature of the latter is the
presence of a venous pulsation, which provides a misleading pulse
oximetry reading.

HOW TO DESCRIBE A MURMUR: Where in cycle/where on
precordium/ radiation/ effect of respiration. RILE: **R** sided murmurs
loudest in **I**nspiration, **L**eft sided loudest in **E**xpiration. NB - a murmur
may not be due to a valve.

HOW TO DESCRIBE A PULSE:
Rate/rhythm/volume/character/tension/vessel wall/equality.

ENDOCARDITIS PROPHYLAXIS

These guidelines change regularly. If in doubt, consult a microbiologist.
INDICATIONS: Prosthetic valves, post-subacute bacterial endocarditis
(SBE) (both are at special risk); post-rheumatic fever mitral regurgitation
(MR), mitral stenosis (MS), aortic stenosis (AS), aortic regurgitation (AR),
bicuspid aortic valve, ventricular septal defect (VSD), atrial septal defect
(ASD), patent ductus arteriosus (PDA). Requirement in mitral leaflet
prolapse is controversial.
DENTAL SURGERY: AMOXYCILLIN 3 g p.o. 4 h preop (or 1g iv at
induction), repeated postop.
- If at special risk: AMOXYCILLIN 1 g + GENTAMICIN 120 mg i.m. or
i.v. at induction, AMOXYCILLIN 500 mg p.o. postop.
- If allergic to penicillin, or had a penicillin more than once in last month:
VANCOMYCIN 1 g (child, 20 mg/kg) over 100 mins + GENTAMICIN
120 mg (2 mg/kg) at induction.
UROLOGY: as for special risk, above. If infected, appropriate to
organism, if identified.
O&G, GI SURGERY: only if at special risk: as for urology.

ANTITHROMBOTIC PROPHYLAXIS

RISK GROUPS: & INCIDENCE OF COMPLICATIONS
LOW RISK: <10% DVT, 0.01% fatal PE
-Surgery <30 mins; no risk factors other than age
-Surgery >30 mins; age <40; no other risk factors
-Minor trauma
MODERATE RISK: 10 - 40% DVT, 0.1 - 1% fatal PE
-Major general, urological, gynae, cardiothoracic, vascular, neuro surgery;
age > 40 or other risk factor
-Major trauma, burns
-Minor surgery or trauma with other risk factor
HIGH RISK: 40 - 80% DVT, 1 - 10% fatal PE
-Surgery of pelvis, hip, lower limb
-Pelvic or abdo surgery for malignancy
-Major surgery with high risk factors
-Lower limb paralysis
-Amputation

OTHER RISK FACTORS: Obesity, varicose veins, immobility,
pregnancy, oestrogens, history of of deep vein thrombosis (DVT) or
pulmonary embolism (PE), thrombophilia, malignancy, cardiac disease,

connective tissue disease. The Concensus paper on which these guidelines did not, strangely, mention smoking as a risk factor.

RECOMMENDATIONS
1. Early mobilisation, all groups.
2. Specific prophylaxis, moderate and high risk groups.
3. Continue prophylaxis until discharge.

METHODS:
- Low dose s/c heparin, 5000u 8 - 12-hourly.
- Adjusted low dose s/c heparin, 3500u 8-hourly, starting 2 days prior to surgery, keeping APTT upper range of normal.
- Low molecular weight heparin.
- Warfarin to keep INR between 2.0 - 2.5.
- Dextran 70
- Graduated compression stockings
- Intermittent pneumatic compression
- Anti-platelet drugs, aspirin or hydroxychloroquine

RECOMMENDATIONS BY SPECIALTY:
General surgery: Medium risk, use low dose heparin or low molecular weight heparin, 12 hourly; high risk, use low dose heparin or low molecular weight heparin, 8 hourly. If contraindicated, then use graduated compression stockings or intermittent pneumatic compression or both.
Urological surgery: Medium risk and high risk use low dose heparin and graduated compression stockings or intermittent pneumatic compression with graduated compression stockings.
Gynaecological surgery: Medium risk use low dose heparin 12 hourly with graduated compression stockings, or intermittent pneumatic compression with graduated compression stockings. In high risk use low dose heparin 8 hourly with graduated compression stockings, or intermittent pneumatic compression with graduated compression stockings.
Cardiac surgery: Medium risk and high risk use anti-platelet drugs, either aspirin or hydroxychloroquine.
Vascular surgery: Medium risk and high risk use low dose heparin.
Neurosurgery: Medium risk and high risk use intermittent pneumatic compression with graduated compression stockings.
Orthopaedic: Elective hip, medium risk and high risk use low molecular weight heparin or adjusted low dose heparin.
Orthopaedic: Hip fractures, medium risk and high risk use adjusted low dose heparin or dextran. If cardiac disease present, use warfarin.
Orthopaedic: Knees, medium risk and high risk use intermittent pneumatic compression with graduated compression stockings.

Combined oral contraceptive: If no other risk factors, do not stop oral contraceptive. In emergency or major elective, use any method.

Pregnancy: If other risk factor present, low dose heparin (and then onto warfarin) from onset of labour and for 6 weeks.

Emergency Caesarean section: If other risk factor present, use low dose heparin until mobile.

From: *Thromboembolic Risk Factors Consensus Group 1992* (*BMJ* **305**, 567-574)

MANAGEMENT OF DIABETES MELLITUS

Beware also renal, vascular, and autonomic complications of the disease when considering a diabetic patient.

PREOPERATIVE MANAGEMENT

The aim is to minimise the metabolic derangement by providing a balance of fluid, calories and insulin, with care to avoid the hazards, which are:

- Hypoglycaemia
- Hyperglycaemia
- Lipolysis
- Proteolysis
- Ketoacidosis
- Dehydration

The preoperative visit must establish three things:

1. Adequacy of blood sugar control.
2. Therapy in use.
3. Degree of multisystem involvement.

NON-INSULIN DEPENDANT DIABETES; MINOR SURGERY

1. Transfer to short-acting agent one week pre-operatively if possible.
2. No tablets on morning of operation. Treat as non-diabetic if BS < 7 mmol/l.
3. Restart tablets with first meal.
4. Give IV glucose with caution if at all.

NON-INSULIN DEPENDANT DIABETES; MAJOR SURGERY

1. As for IDDM. See below.
2. Once eating: tds soluble insulin (Actrapid) 8 - 12u before each meal. Revert to tablets once insulin > 20u/day.

INSULIN-DEPENDANT DIABETES: ALBERTI REGIME
1. Convert to soluble insulin over 3 days.
2. No insulin in morning of operation.
3. Set up infusion 500 ml 10% Dextrose with 10u Actrapid and 10 mmol KCl; run at 100 ml/hour (adult). Check BS and K^+ every 2 hours and adjust as necessary. This entails discarding the entire bag and starting again; this is a major criticism of the regime, as in addition to waste, it makes accurate recording of fluid intake difficult.
4. Stop infusion when oral feeding recommenced, go to tds Actrapid (Daily dose + 20% if infected, + 20% if on steroids).

INSULIN-DEPENDANT DIABETES: CONTINUOUS INSULIN AND DEXTROSE
1. Convert to soluble insulin.
2. Commence infusion 10% Dextrose from starvation, at 100 ml/hour (adult).
3. Soluble insulin by infusion; there are a number of "sliding scales" available. This is an example.
4. Start at 0.5 - 1.0 units/hour.

Blood Glucose	Infusion (Units/hour)
<5.0	Off, give 25 mls 50% Dextrose, once >7, restart at 0.3 - 0.6
5.0 - 7.0	Decrease by 0.3
7.1 - 10.0	No change
10.1 - 14.0	Increase by 0.3
>14.0	Increase by 0.5

OBESITY

The Body Mass index (BMI) = weight (kg)/height (m)^2. Normal is 20 - 25; 25 - 30 is overweight, and over 30 is obesity. This is an actuarial index (also known as the Quetelet index) and is used to identify that group which is at greater risk of:

1. Hypertension, right ventricular hypertrophy, ischaemic heart disease and increased oxygen consumption.

2. Decreased respiratory compliance and reduced FRC.

3. Gastro-intestinal reflux and hiatus hernia.

4. Endocrine problems: glucose tolerance often impaired, sometimes to the point of frank diabetes.

5. Altered pharmacokinetics: increased volume of distribution for lipid-soluble drugs, e.g. induction agents.

HYPERTENSION

Condition must be optimised and medication must be continued up to and including the morning of operation. Beware co-existing silent ischaemia which occurs in the morning, in the elderly, in diabetics and is three times as common as angina. It is suggested by fatigue, arrhythmia and acute left ventricular failure.

A β-blocker e.g. metoprolol 50 mg may be given as a premedicant if the patient is not already on such a drug, as it reduces rate, reduces contractility and is antidysrhythmic.

Critical periods are intubation and extubation, incision and visceral handling, as well as periods of changes in circulating volume.
(See also under Initial Assessment, but remember Goldman did not include hypertension in the Cardiac Risk Index).

MALIGNANCY

Specific problems include:

1. Cachexia and poor nutritional state.

2. Low proteins and enhanced effect of protein-bound drugs.

3. Anaemia and cardiac failure.

4. Hypercalcaemia; levels over 3.75mmol/l may be reduced by phosphate infusion (or infusion of biphosphonates) in an emergency, or by oral phosphate, steroids (although there is now some doubt over the efficacy of steroids in malignancy) and rehydration if time permits. It is

hypocalcaemia which causes tetany, and this may happen if hypercalcaemia is corrected too rapidly.

5. Eaton-Lambert syndrome and susceptibility to neuromuscular blockade.

Notes

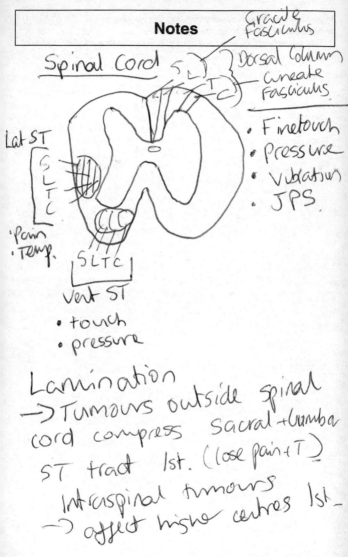

Spinal Cord

Gracile Fasciculus

Dorsal Column
Cuneate Fasciculus

- Fine touch
- Pressure
- Vibration
- JPS

Lat ST
[S L T C]

- Pain
- Temp.

[S L T C]
Vent ST

- touch
- pressure

Lamination
→ Tumours outside spinal cord compress sacral + lumbar ST tract 1st. (lose pain + T)
Intraspinal tumours → affect higher centres 1st.

Practical anaesthesia

RECORD OF GENERAL ANAESTHESIA

This is the author's personal way of recording a general anaesthetic, and the way I teach new trainees to think and record their thoughts. As ever, it is intended to remind and prevent omissions.

INDUCTION:
- Venous access, on non-dominant arm for preference.

AIRWAY:
- Means of control; tracheal tube, laryngeal mask or mask and airway.
- Cords sprayed with lignocaine?
- Gas entry, confirmed in the anaesthetic room and again in theatre, by capnography as method of choice.
- PACK? Put in capitals if you have placed a pharyngeal pack, to remind you to remove it at the end of the case.
- Record the Cormack & Lehane view at intubation, so the next colleague attending the patient knows what to expect:

    I: Glottis in sight, complete.

    II: Glottis in sight, but only the posterior part.

    III: Epiglottis only seen.

    IV: Nothing seen. The benefit to a colleague reviewing your

notes if you have recorded this is obvious.

MAINTENANCE OF ANAESTHESIA:
- Spontaneous respiration (SR) or intermittent positive pressure ventilation (IPPV)?
- Machine type; record if circle used.
- Gases: record inspired oxygen fraction (FiO_2), fresh gas flow, and the volatile agent used.
- Ventilation: record minute ventilation (V_E), tidal volume (V_T) frequency of ventilation (f) and patient system pressure (PSP).

GUEDEL: Described stages of anaesthesia in gaseous induction using ether.

First stage: Analgesia; to loss of consciousness.

Second stage: Excitement; to onset of automatic breathing.

Third stage: To respiratory paralysis.

> Plane 1: To cessation of eye movement.
> Plane 2: To start of intercostal paralysis.
> Plane 3: To completion of intercostal paralysis.
> Plane 4: To diaphragmatic paralysis.

Fourth stage: overdose.

POSITION:

- Record the patient position, taping of the eyes, and protection of pressure points such as elbows and the peroneal nerve at the knee.

ADJUNCTIVE ANAESTHESIA:

- Regional; epidural, brachial plexus or femoral, for example.
- Infiltration, by surgeon or anaesthetist.

OTHER TECHNIQUES:

- Naso- or oro-gastric tube
- Pneumoperitoneum
- Table tilt
- Warming blanket
- Blood warmer
- Cell salvage
- Aprotinin

MONITORS:

These may be divided into those which monitor the condition of the patient, and those which monitor the equipment. One device, the capnograph, monitors both.

Patient	Equipment
Non-invasive blood pressure	Patient system pressure
ECG	Disconnection
SpO$_2$	O$_2$ failure
P$_E$CO$_2$	Gas analysis
Peripheral nerve stimulator (PNS)	
Temperature	
Central venous pressure	
Invasive blood pressure	
Pulmonary artery catheter	

BLOOD LOSS:

From swabs and from suction.

FLUIDS ADMINISTERED:

These should be timed entries, so that you can demonstrate that you responded to a drop in blood pressure, for example. The record of fluid administered must also appear on the patient's drug chart, or it may otherwise not be included in the fluid balance for the day of theatre. Bearing in mind that up to 3 litres may be administered during the course of a long, but routine, laparotomy, this volume is significant. Fluid overload is a frequent cause of admission to the intensive care unit.

REVERSAL:

Admit to doxapram if you used it.

POSTOPERATIVE INSTRUCTIONS:

- Oxygen: Flow rate and duration required. Hypoxia occurs at night, and up to the third postoperative night.
- Analgesia: Intramuscular opiate, patient controlled analgesia (PCA), or epidural, by infusion or top-up.
- Fluids to be administered, venous access, and how long the access should be maintained. Overnight for tonsillectomy with adenoidectomy, for example.
- Observations.
  See Postoperative Management section at the end of this chapter.

MACHINE CHECKLIST

OXYGEN ANALYSER:
Calibrate to room air, and to 100% oxygen.

GAS SUPPLIES:
1. Disconnect pipelines and turn off cylinders.
2. Open all rotameters.
3. Turn on each O_2 cylinder and operate rotameter; set at 5 L/min;
          OBSERVE-   Analyser reads 100%.
4. Repeat for N_2O. Leave O_2 on 5 L/min.
5. Turn off O_2 cylinder and void system via flush valve
          OBSERVE- O_2 gauge fall.
                              Audible alarm.
                              Prevention of hypoxic mixture.
6. Connect O_2 pipeline.
          OBSERVE- O_2 flow restored.
                              Audible alarm silenced.
7. Perform "Tug test"
          OBSERVE-   400 kPa indicated on gauge.
8. Repeat 6&7 for N_2O.
9. Turn off all rotameters, operate O_2 flush;
          OBSERVE-   No drop in pipeline pressure.
                              100% on O_2 analyser.

VAPORISERS:
1. Secure position on backbar, free dial movement.
2. Flow is in correct direction.
3. Vaporiser full, with the correct agent, filling port closed.
4. If pressure relief valve (PRV) fitted, set O_2 to 6 L/min, occlude common gas outlet (CGO)
          OBSERVE-   No leak.
                              Dip in bobbin
5. Repeat with vaporiser turned on. Unseated vaporisers are a major cause of awareness.

BREATHING SYSTEM:
1. Correct configuration, no leaks, no obstructions.
2. "Push and twist" all conical fittings.
3. Expiratory valve opens and closes.
4. Bain attachment; perform occlusion test, observe bobbin drop; use oxygen flush, observe venturi effect collapse the bag. The vulnerable point is the connection of the fresh gas flow to the inner tube. This can be confirmed visually as well.
5. Circle; confirm function of unidirectional valves.

VENTILATOR:
1. Make it work.
2. Occlude patient port;
             OBSERVE-   PRV Function
3. Confirm that disconnect warning alarm works.
4. Ensure that alternative means of ventilation is available.

SUCTION:
This is what candidates forget in the exam, apparantly.

SPARE LARYNGOSCOPES AND TRACHEAL TUBES

DRUGS DRAWN UP:
1. SUXAMETHONIUM
2. ATROPINE
3. EPHEDRINE, whenever a regional block is used.

Adapted from: *Association of Anaesthetists*

FAILED RAPID SEQUENCE INTUBATION DRILL

You must have an immediate action drill for this eventuality. It was first described by Tunstall in connection with failed obstetric intubation, and has been modified many times since. It is also appropriate for other situations where the airway is at risk of soiling with gastric contents. Oxygenation is paramount.

NO SECOND DOSE SUXAMETHONIUM
DO NOT RENDER HYPOXIC

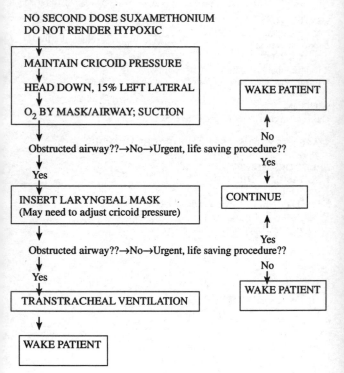

MAINTAIN CRICOID PRESSURE

HEAD DOWN, 15% LEFT LATERAL

O_2 BY MASK/AIRWAY; SUCTION

Obstructed airway??→No→Urgent, life saving procedure??

Yes

No

WAKE PATIENT

Yes

INSERT LARYNGEAL MASK
(May need to adjust cricoid pressure)

CONTINUE

Yes

Obstructed airway??→No→Urgent, life saving procedure??

Yes

No

WAKE PATIENT

TRANSTRACHEAL VENTILATION

WAKE PATIENT

EQUIPMENT

CYLINDERS AND GAS SUPPLIES

The supply for machines in most operating theatres in the developed world is by pipeline, with cylinders as back-up. The gases are delivered at 4 Bar (420 kPa, 60 psi). Oxygen comes from a Vacuum Insulated Evaporator (VIE) at -183^0c and nitrous oxide from a manifold of cylinders. After heat exchanging and pressure reduction, they enter the theatre at terminal outlets, where a Schraeder probe leads to a gas-specific hose, which in turn connects to a Non-Interchangeable Screw Thread (NIST) at the anaesthetic machine. There are either one or two pressure regulators (also called pressure reducing valves) within the machine (the number depends on the manufacturer) after which there is a pressure relief valve which operates at 800 kPa (8 Bar, 120 psi) in order to protect the machine from damage. On the back bar, where the vaporisers are situated, there is a pressure relief valve which operates at 42 kPa (6 psi), which protects the patient.

There is also an oxygen failure device, which diverts the remaining gas through an audible alarm before opening the system to room air.

Cylinders for anaesthetic gases are made of molybdenum steel. Some may be fitted with a Wood's metal fusible plug in the valve block which melts at low temperature, with the intention of avoiding explosion if the cylinder is exposed to fire or other high temperature. 1 in every 100 is tested to destruction, and every one is tested to 10% over the working pressure every three years. The tare is the weight of the cylinder empty. Knowledge of the tare allows a full cylinder to be distinguished from an empty one.

MARKINGS:

OXYGEN: Black with white shoulders, sizes C-J, plus AF.

NITROUS OXIDE: Blue with blue shoulders, sizes C-G

ENTONOX: Blue with blue and white shoulders, sizes D, F and G.

AIR: Grey with black and white shoulders, sizes E-J.

CARBON DIOXIDE: Grey with grey shoulders, sizes C,E and F.

CYCLOPROPANE: Orange with orange shoulders, size B only.

HELIUM: Dark orange, sizes D and F.

SIZES:
Size B: Tare 1.6 kg, volume 180 litres, cyclopropane only.
Size C: Tare 2 kg, volume 170 litres O_2, 450 litres N_2O.
Size D: Tare 3.4 kg, volume 340 litres O_2, 900 litres N_2O, 500 litres
Entonox.
Size E: Tare 5.4 kg, volume 680 litres O_2, 1800 litres N_2O.
Size F: Tare 14.5 kg, volume 1360 litres O_2, 3600 litres N_2O, 2000 litres
Entonox.
Size AF: Tare 9.9 kg, volume 1360 litres O_2 only.
Size G: Tare 34.5 kg, volume 3400 litres O_2, 9000 litres N_2O, 5000 litres
Entonox.
Size J: Tare 68.9 kg, volume 6800 litres O_2, 6400 litres air.

PIN INDEX:

Oxygen 2-5	Nitrous oxide 3-5
Cyclopropane 3-6	Entonox 7
Air 1-5	

PHYSICAL CHARACTERISTICS OF GASES
A vapour is a substance in a gaseous state at a temperature and pressure
close to those at which it would liquefy. The critical temperature is the
temperature above which a vapour cannot be kept in the gaseous state by
the effect of pressure alone. This does not mean that the substance, if kept
in a cylinder above the critical temperature, will explode; what it means is
that the contents of that cylinder will be in the gaseous phase. It would
otherwise be unsafe to store nitrous oxide in the tropics. The critical
pressure is the pressure required to liquefy a gas at its critical temperature.

Gas	Critical Temperature	Critical Pressure	Cylinder Pressure
CO_2	31°c	72.85 bar	50 bar
N_2O	36.5°c	72.6 bar	44 bar
O_2	-118.4°c	50.14 bar	134.7 bar

GAUGES:
The French gauge is the circumference in millimetres x 3.
The wire gauge is 20 - 20(log ext. diameter), roughly the number of wires
that size which will pass through a 1" ring.

VOLATILE AGENT CONSUMPTION:
This may be calculated from

(flow x concentration)$_{STP}$ x $\dfrac{MW}{22.4 \times SG}$

STP = standard temperature and pressure.
MW = molecular weight of the volatile.
SG = Specific gravity of the volatile.

FLOWMETERS:
These are commonly known as rotameters, although this is a trade term. Each is individually calibrated and lined with a very thin film of gold to prevent static making the bobbin adhere to the side and a spurious reading result. They are therefore the most expensive component of an anaesthetic machine.

Part of the flowmeter	Cross section	Type of flow	Important gas characteristic
Bottom	Tubular	Laminar	Viscosity dependant
Top	Orificial	Turbulent	Density dependant

CLASSIFICATION OF VAPORISERS AND BREATHING SYSTEMS

CONWAY CLASSIFICATION
This is the classic way of describing a breathing system.
- OPEN: No exclusion of ambient air, no confinement of exhaled gases.
- SEMI-OPEN: Partial exclusion of ambient air, partial confinement of exhaled gases; an example is the Schimmelbusch mask.
- SEMI-CLOSED: Fully bounded system, with provision for gas overflow; examples include the Bain and Magill attachments.
- CLOSED: A fully bounded circuit, no overflow of exhaled gases; the only example is a circle with the expiratory valve screwed down and a minimum fresh gas flow.

DORSCH & DORSCH
This is a way of describing a vaporiser in an exam.
- METHOD FOR REGULATING CONCENTRATION: Variable bypass or measured flow.
- METHOD OF VAPORISATION: Flowover or bubble-through.
- LOCATION: In or out of circle. A plenum system is one where the pressure within is greater than the pressure without. Most contemporary vaporisers are plenum vaporisers, and cannot be used as drawover vaporisers as the resistance to flow is too great.
- TEMPERATURE COMPENSATION: None, supplied heat or bimetallic strip.
- SPECIFICITY: For different vapours.

MAPLESON CLASSIFICATION

This is the classical way of describing a breathing attachment. Few of them are circular, so describing them as circuits is inappropriate.

In all cases, the arrow indicates the fresh gas entry and the bar indicates the adjustable pressure relief valve. Mapleson is a professor of the Physics of Anaesthesia.

MAPLESON A: The Magill attachment is the classical exmple of this.

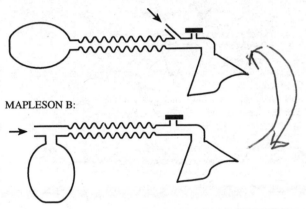

MAPLESON B:

MAPLESON C: The Waters to-and-fro, used for ventilation while transferring patients and for physiotherapy on the Intensive Care Unit.

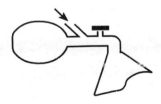

MAPLESON D: The Bain attachment is functionally a Mapleson D arrangement.

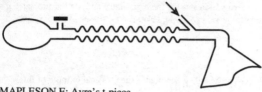

MAPLESON E: Ayre's t-piece.

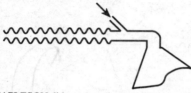

MAPLESON did not describe F, but the expression is much used to describe Jackson-Rees' modification of Ayres' t-piece:

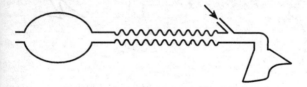

GAS AND VENTILATION

FRESH GAS FLOWS
FOR SPONTANEOUS RESPIRATION:
>Bain (Mapleson D): 2 - 3 x minute ventilation.
>Magill (Mapleson A): Alveolar ventilation.

FOR CONTROLLED VENTILATION:
>Bain: 70 mls/kg/min to keep $PaCO_2$ 5.3 kPa..

>Ayre's t-piece: 2 - 3 x minute ventilation, and in any case more than 4 l/min. The volume of the limb must exceed tidal volume or dilution of fresh gas with room air occurs.

FOR CIRCLES: Low flow is defined as less than 3 l/min. To perform this safely, most would advocate the use of agent and carbon dioxide monitoring.

VENTILATION VALUES
In the awake resting state these may be calculated as follows:

Body weight (kg)	Minute volume, V_E (mls)	Tidal volume, V_T(mls)
2	480	14 - 16
3	600	17 - 24
7	1,000	50 - 60
10	1,680	80

(handwritten annotations beside table: (16)× 30/min; (20)× 30/min; (50)× 20; ×20/min)

V_E = minute ventilation
V_T = tidal volume

THEREAFTER: V_T = 8 mls/kg
V_E = 4,000 mls for 30 kgBW
= 5,600 mls for 70 kgBW

PRESSURE CONVERSIONS

Different machines use different units of pressure. They may also use different units from those used in physiology. Converting between them all is a problem, but a few calculations may help.

1 atm = 1 bar = 1,000 millibars.
         = 101 kPa = 101,000 N/m^2
            ≈15 psi.
                     = 760 mmHg = 760 Torr.
1 kPa ≈ 10 cmH$_2$O = 100 mmH$_2$O

So;   100 kPa   = 15 psi
              1 kPa   ≈ 0.15 psi
              1 psi   ≈ 6.66 kPa

And;   100 kPa   = 760 mmHg
              1 kPa   = 7.6 mmHg
              10 mmHg = 1.32 kPa

Regarding the sitting patient: 1 cmH$_2$0 = 0.76 mmHg. Thus the perfusion pressure of the head falls by 0.76 mmHg from the recorded pressure at chest level for every 1 cm that the head is above the level of the chest. This is of relevance in surgery in the sitting position, especially if hypotension has been induced.

MONITORING DEFAULT VALUES

The default value is the alarm setting which is set at the factory and comes into operation when the machine is turned on from cold. These are some examples; the point is that the default values may be inappropriately set and may not offer the sort of protection against excessively high or low readings that the anaesthetist may have expected when he or she sets up at the start of a list.

Ohmeda Saturation Monitor	
High O_2	not set
Low O_2	90%
High pulse	not set
Low pulse	not set
S&W Diascope	
High pulse	240
Low pulse	0
Critikon Dinamapp (Models vary)	
High mean arterial pressure	140
Low mean arterial pressure	50
Low heart rate	40 - no recording
Datex Capnomac	
High P_ECO_2	7.0%
Low P_ECO_2	3.0
Inspired P_ECO_2	1%
Low FiO_2	18%
High FiO_2	not set
High N_2O	85%
High volatile concentration	5.0%
Low volatile concentration	0 %
Apnoea	25 sec
OAV 7750 ventilator	
Low minute volume	Not set
Low FiO_2	23%

Datascope passport	
High heart rate	160
Low heart rate	40
High SpO_2	100%
Low SpO_2	85%
High systolic	200 mmHg
Low systolic	70 mmHg
Low respiratory rate	5
High respiratory rate	50
Low P_ECO_2	3 kPa
High P_ECO_2	9 kPa

HARVARD MINIMUM MONITORING STANDARDS

These were implemented to reduce malpractice premiums but have become accepted as the basis of good anaesthetic practice since then.

1. Presence of anaesthetist throughout procedure and until patient fully recovered. AN
2. ECG. C
3. Blood pressure and heart rate measured and recorded every 5 minutes. C
4. Observation of ventilation: Movement of the bag, or monitoring breath sounds, or end-tidal CO_2. B
5. Observation of the circulation: Palpation of pulse, or SpO_2. C
6. Disconnection alarm. A
7. Measurement of FiO_2. A

The ability to record patient temperature was added as a footnote.

Anaesthetist

A — Alarm (disconnect)
— FiO_2

B — ventilation — obs
BS
Capnograph

C — ECG
Obs circuln — Pulse
SpO_2
BP/HR measured + recorded.

CAPNOGRAPHY

Capnography is possibly the single most useful monitor in general anaesthetic practice.

Definitions:

A CAPNOGRAPH is a device which records and displays the CO_2 concentration.

A CAPNOGRAM is a graphical plot of CO_2 as a function of time.

A CAPNOMETER is an instrument for measuring the numerical concentration of CO_2. Thus, all capnographs are capnometers, but a capnometer need not display a capnogram.

REALTIME: A capnogram waveform displayed at 12.5 mm/sec, demonstrating fine detail and sudden changes in morphology.

TREND: A capnogram waveform displayed at 25 mm/min, demonstrating gradual changes over time.

DELAY TIME: The sum of the transit time and the rise time.

TRANSIT TIME: The time taken for a sample to be delivered from the point of interest to the analyser.

RISE TIME: The time taken by the capnographic cell to register from 10% to 90% of a step change after the sample has entered the measuring chamber. The latter is also known as the response time, and is important as it must be less than the time taken for one breath.

MAINSTREAM: Where the analysing cell is interposed in the breathing system. These do not cause turbulent flow in the breathing system nor do they extract gas from it (both of importance in paediatric anaesthesia) and they have a short delay time, but they are vulnerable to being dropped and damaged. They are also heavy and difficult to support when using a mask. They heat up.

SIDESTREAM: Where a continuous sample is drawn at the rate of 150 ml/min from the breathing system to be analysed within the machine. This is the more common arrangement, but the gas needs to be scavenged, or returned to the system if a circle is in use. Condensation forms and a water-trap is needed.

INFRARED ANALYSIS: This uses absorption of infrared light.

MASS SPECTROMETRY: This uses deviation of ions in a magnetic field.

RAMAN SCATTERING: This uses bombardment, and scattering, of light particles.

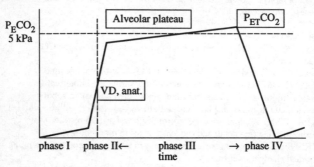

PATTERNS ASSOCIATED WITH PARTICULAR DISORDERS:

- Malignant hyperpyrexia: High peak PCO_2.
- Chronic airways disease: Slow upstroke, wide $P(a\text{-}ET)CO_2$ gradient.
- Defective valves in a circle system: Raised baseline with oscillations.
- CO_2 rebreathing: Raised baseline, with oscillations in phase IV.
- Circulatory arrest: Progressive diminution in amplitude.
- Oesophageal intubation: Even with carbonated drink in stomach, less than 6 deflections will be seen. Thereafter, the tube cannot be in the trachea if no CO_2 is detected, unless circulatory arrest has occurred.
- Airway obstruction: Slow ascent phase II.
- Recovery from neuromuscular blockade during positive pressure ventilation: Clefts are seen during phase III.

NITROUS OXIDE ABSORPTION

- Initially: 400 ml/min
- After 1 hr: 75 ml/min
- After 3 hr: 20 ml/min

Absorption is governed by a process of two time constants, of 25 and 500 minutes respectively.

OXIMETRY

This may be pulse oximetry (in vivo) or bench oximetry (haemolysed sample, in vitro; co-oximetry). The advantage of bench oximetry is that it can differentiate between different species of haemoglobin (e.g. COHb, MetHb).

PULSE OXIMETRY

Light is transmitted across a digit or extremity from an LED to a photodiode, at two wavelengths, 660 and 940 nm. Reduced Hb absorbs better at 660 nm and oxygenated Hb at 940 nm. They are the same at the isobestic point (803 nm). The non-pulsatile component of the signal (venous blood, unless a venous pulse is present, e.g. tricuspid incompetence) is subtracted by a microprocessor, leaving the arterial component to be measured.

It is most accurate above 90% saturation, and much less accurate below 70%. They are calibrated against healthy volunteers, which makes calibration to values below 70% ethically unacceptable. Problems leading to inaccuracies include:
1. Vasoconstriction.
2. Venous engorgement and pulsation.
3. Bile, dyes.
4. Abnormal Hb (especially COHb, which gives a spuriously high reading).
5. Motion.
6. Ambient light.
7. Diathermy.

NEUROMUSCULAR MONITORING

Nerve stimulator: delivers 50 mA for 0.2 - 1.0 msec; requires 50 - 300 V.

TWITCH-TETANUS-TWITCH: This distinguishes the *type* of block; four patterns are observed.
1.   Normal; symmetrical twitches followed by sustained tetanic contraction; no post-tetanic facilitation (PTF).
2.   Total block; no response.
3.   Partial depolarising block; weak but symmetrical twitches, sustained tetanic contraction, no PTF.
4.   Partial non-depolarising block; weak twitches, fade on tetanic stimulus, post-tetanic facilitation.

TRAIN OF FOUR: This distinguishes the *degree* of block. It is possible to use the count, or the ratio of force of 4th to 1st twitch (T4:T1).

Count 1,2,3	75% block
Count 1,2	80% block
Count 1	90% block
Count 0	100% block.

POST-TETANIC TWITCH COUNT: This determines the *reversibility* of a block; the device delivers 50 Hz for 5 sec, then 1 Hz, counting detectable twitches. Reversal is possible if count is greater than 10.

DOUBLE BURST: This uses 3 pairs of 50 Hz pulses separated by 0.75 sec. It assesses *recovery* from block, displaying the T1:T4 ratio.

ENDOBRONCHIAL TUBES

INDICATIONS FOR USE
1. Absolute indications (these are usually anaesthetic reasons):
      a. Rupture or fistula.
      b. Massive haemorrhage.
      c. Bronchoplastic procedures: one-lung transplant.
2. Relative indications (usually surgical):
      a. Lung resection.
      b. Oesophageal surgery.

IDENTIFICATION OF TYPES
The smallest available are 26 FG. Observe and describe: lumens, cuffs, pilot balloons, oropharyngeal and bronchial curves, orifices (especially if in a cuff), and suction orifices.

This is a key for identification of different tubes in use.

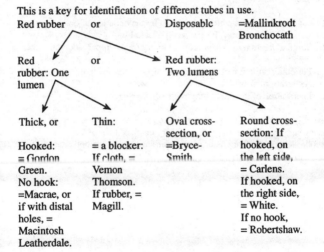

Red rubber   or   Disposable   =Mallinkrodt
                                          Bronchocath

Red rubber: One lumen   or   Red rubber: Two lumens

Thick, or   Thin: Oval cross-section, or   Round cross-section: If

Hooked:
= Gordon Green.
No hook:
=Macrae, or if with distal holes, = Macintosh Leatherdale.

Thin:
= a blocker:
If cloth, = Vemon Thomson.
If rubber, = Magill.

Oval cross-section, or
=Bryce-Smith

Round cross-section: If hooked, on the left side, = Carlens.
If hooked, on the right side, = White.
If no hook, = Robertshaw.

CONFIRMATION OF PLACEMENT

Fibreoptic examination is the definitive method.
The key is to **isolate** the upper, operative lung and to **ventilate** the dependant, lower lung.

1. Inflate tracheal cuff: hear BS over both lungfields.
2. Inflate bronchial cuff, deflate tracheal cuff: hear sounds only on bronchially-intubated side.
3. Then ventilate each side separately.
4. Repeat after patient movement.

The surgeon will invite you to "let the lung down". To do this, clamp the tracheal lumen (red marking) and remove the bung from the top of its tube; the bronchially-intubated (blue marking) tube will now ventilate the dependant lung, and the upper lung will be isolated and should deflate. If there is a leak around the bronchial cuff, however, the upper lung may reinflate.

The considerable shunt which is imposed by the deflation of one lung must be monitored by oximetry. It may be alleviated by:

1. Surgical ligation of the pulmonary artery on the upper side: this closes the shunt.
2. Periodic reinflation of the operative, upper lung, with the surgeon's cooperation.
3. Insufflation of the upper lung with 100% oxygen.

Use of pressure-volume and flow-volume loops displayed on a monitor during surgery will identify the secondary displacement of an endobronchial tube from its original position, because the appearance of the loops will alter with time.

REGIONAL ANAESTHESIA

LOCAL ANAESTHETIC AGENTS

Procaine, cocaine and amethocaine are esters, and are metabolised by plasma cholinesterase; the others are amides, which are metabolised in the liver. They are prepared in acid solution (pH 4-5) of Ringers solution as water-soluble hydrochloride salts. After injection the uncharged base enters the axoplasm where it combines with H^+ ions to adopt the charged ionic form which is active.

- Potency is related to lipid solubility;
- Duration is proportional to protein binding;
- Rate of onset is proportional to the proximity of the agent's pKa to tissue pH.

The pKa of all esters is between 8.5 and 9.0; the pKa of all amides is between 7.6 and 7.9, with the exception of bupivacaine, which has a pKa of 8.1. They are all weak bases.

SAFE MAXIMAL DOSES

These may be doubled with addition of a vasoconstrictor. Absorption is very dependant on the route of administration; intercostal local anaesthetic is absorbed most rapidly, followed by topical administration.

Bupivacaine	2 mg/kg body weight.
Lignocaine	3 mg/kg body weight.
Prilocaine	6 mg/kg body weight.

Signs of toxicity appear first in the central nervous system with reduced level of consciousness, circumoral tingling and, eventually convulsions. The principal cardiovascular side effect is of ventricular arrhythmia, which may be refractory to usual treatment. The CC/CNS (cardiac collapse to CNS side effects) ratio is 7:1 for lignocaine but only 4:1 for bupivacaine. The treatment of local-anaesthetic induced arrhythmia is bretylium, 7 mg/kg body weight, or phenytoin, 5 mg/kg body weight. The latter is advocated in paediatric circumstances by authorities at Great Ormond Street.

PROCEDURE
This is a template for describing any regional technique.

PATIENT suitability and consent.
CANNULATE a vein.
RESUSCITATION kit available.
POSITION of patient.
LANDMARKS of nerve or space, and tissues penetrated.
NEEDLE size and length; most needles will be 22G, other than for the eye and in obstetrics. Pencil points are best for spinals. Short bevels cause more damage if the enter a nerve but are less likely to do so.
ENDPOINT bone, distance, loss of resistance. The use of a nerve stimulator with an insulated needle will identify the nerve group to be blocked, as well as others to be avoided; for example, the phrenic nerve when performing an interscalene block.
ASPIRATE to exclude intravascular or subarachnoid placement of needle or catheter.
DEPTH and LENGTH of catheter for epidurals.
INJECTION volume and concentration.
WATCH for effects and complications, notably;
        1. Inadvertent subarachnoid, subdural;
        2. Inadvertent intravascular injection.
ADRENALINE: 10 ml of 1:100,000 every 10 minutes when using Halothane; this is 0.1 mg.
In other situations the maximum dose is 0.5 mg.

COMBINED SUBARACHNOID-EPIDURAL FOR OBSTETRICS

The following are procedures followed at Queen Charlotte's and Chelsea Hospital.

AMBULATORY EPIDURAL FOR LABOUR

The aims are to provide analgesia but without compromising motor function, so as to permit ambulation and improve maternal satisfaction.

CONTRAINDICATIONS

1. Refusal
2. Bleeding diathesis (but not aspirin)
3. Severe PET: Platelets < 80,000, fitting, LVF.
4. Back surgery (relative)
5. Sepsis
6. Valvular or other heart disease
7. Raised intracranial pressure

PRELOAD:

500 ml Hartmann's solution BP (HSBP).

PROCEDURE:

Explanation to patient, positioning, blood pressure and foetal monitoring.

1. Use 16G Tuohy needle to locate epidural space, using loss of resistance to either air or saline.
2. Pass a 27G, 12 cm spinal needle via Tuohy to subarachnoid space, inject:

- Bupivacaine 2.5 mg (1.0 ml of 0.25%)
- Fentanyl 25 mcg
- Saline 0.5 ml

Withdraw spinal needle, thread epidural catheter. No epidural drugs at this stage.

Observe for 20 minutes:

> BP
>
> Level   Sensory - both top and bottom of block.
>   Motor
>   Sympathetic

If appropriate, ambulate

If unilateral, turn to unblocked side, give 5 ml of epidural mixture (see below); then further 10 ml in supine position; thereafter, resite catheter. No second subarachnoid injection.

If inadequate, give epidural injection.
If severe rectal pressure, give fentanyl 100 mcg in 10 ml saline, via epidural.

FIRST EPIDURAL INJECTION

The subarachnoid block wears off abruptly at about 90 minutes. For the first epidural dose, no test dose is necessary, as it has been shown that the therapeutic top-up dose, if given deliberately into the subarachnoid space, produces a block to the high thoracic segments but no further. The first top-up consists of 15 ml of mixture as below, with subsequent doses of 10 ml as required. The mixture consists of:

- Bupivacaine 50 mg (10 ml of 0.5%)
- Fentanyl 100 mcg
- Made up to 50 ml with saline,

and represents:

- Bupivacaine 1.0 mg/ml (0.1% bupivacaine).
- Fentanyl 2.0 mcg/ml.

REGIONAL BLOCK FOR LOWER SEGMENT CAESAREAN SECTION

Preservation of motor function is not appropriate. Aim to achieve sensory block from T4 to S5.

ANTACIDS:
Give 150 mg ranitidine on the night before (for elective cases), repeated 1½ hours preoperatively with 10 mg metoclopramide. Give sodium citrate 0.3M 30 ml in theatre.

MONITORING:
ECG, SpO2, blood pressure; cardiotocograph and a midwife to monitor the fetus.

PRELOAD:
This consists of 1,000 ml Hartmann's solution (restrict to 500 ml if pre-eclamptic), then 1,000 ml Hartmann's with ephedrine 60 mg (not in pre-eclampsia) during procedure, with increments of ephedrine 6 mg to keep systolic pressure greater than 100 mmHg. Ephedrine is especially useful on turning to left tilt from left lateral, immediately prior to skin preparation, when hypotension is otherwise commonly seen.

PROCEDURE: ELECTIVE LSCS
Combined spinal-epidural (CSE) technique as above, using 2 ml of 0.5% hyperbaric bupivacaine for subarachnoid block, with the addition of fentanyl 25 mcg if appropriate. For post-operative pain relief, use lignocaine, 10 ml of 2%, via catheter, followed by diamorphine, 2.5 mg in 10 ml saline, in recovery. This is augmented by diclofenac 100 mg PR stat repeated for three days, with co-codamol or other compound oral analgesic as required.
Other drugs to be drawn up:
- Metoclopramide 10 mg
- Cefuroxime 750 mg
- Syntocinon 10 u.

PROCEDURE: EMERGENCY LSCS:

Place mother in full left lateral position. Give oxygen by facemask.
Consider salbutamol for tocolysis, remind midwife to turn off syntocinon.
Extend the existing epidural with:

- Bupivacaine, 10 ml of 0.5% with adrenaline 1:200.000 with
- Lignocaine, 10 ml of 2%, and
- Fentanyl, 100 mcg

If unsuccessful, or epidural not sited:
Immediate spinal block:

- Bupivacaine, 2.5 ml of hyperbaric 0.5%, with
- Fentanyl 25 mcg, but beware risk of high block.

If in pain during procedure:

- Give entonox, then epidural lignocaine, 10 ml of 2% with
  diamorphine 2.5 mg.

Postoperative analgesia, and other drugs, as above.

PERIBULBAR BLOCK

POSITION: Supine.
LANDMARKS: Medial canthus, at caruncle; apply 1% amethocaine to conjunctiva.
NEEDLE : 25 G, 25 mm short bevel, perpendicular to skin, parrallel to septum.
ENDPOINT: Just short of end of needle.
INJECTION: 8 ml 2% prilocaine with hyalase 500u.

INTERSCALENE BLOCK

POSITION: Supine, arm by side, invite to sniff or to lift head slightly off pillow to identify interscalene groove.
LANDMARKS: Cricoid cartilage, level of C6; interscalene groove. This block lends itself to being performed with a nerve stimulator.
NEEDLE : Insulated 25 G.
ENDPOINT: Eliciting twitches in arm.
INJECTION: 20 ml 0.5% bupivacaine.

AXILLARY BLOCK

POSITION: Supine, hand abducted, elbow flexed, hand pronated.
LANDMARKS: Pulsation of axillary artery within sheath.
NEEDLE : Insulated 25G.
ENDPOINT: Eliciting twitching in arm. Some recommend transfixion of the artery.
INJECTION: 20 ml 0.5% bupivacaine.

STELLATE GANGLION BLOCK

POSITION: Supine.
LANDMARKS: Transverse process of C6: Chassaignac's tubercle.
NEEDLE : Short bevel, 25G.
ENDPOINT: Bone; withdraw fractionally.
INJECTION: 5 ml 2% lignocaine.

THREE-IN-ONE BLOCK

POSITION: Supine.
LANDMARKS: Immediately lateral to the pulsation of the femoral artery.
NEEDLE : Short bevel, 22 G, 5 cm.
ENDPOINT: Paraesthesia in femoral distribution.
INJECTION: Patient height (inches)/3 in ml of 0.5% bupivacaine.

POSTOPERATIVE MANAGEMENT

RECOVERY INSTRUCTIONS

When handing over to the recovery staff, the following are the essential items of information:

- Nature of operation and duration of anaesthetic;
- Whether intubated or not;
- Analgesia provided so far.

The instructions to recovery staff may be considered under the following headings:

1. Timing and frequency of observations required.
2. Oxygen therapy to be given, and duration.
3. Duration of monitoring of oxyhaemoglobin saturation.
4. Respiratory rate which is acceptable.
5. Heart rate and rhythm which is acceptable.
6. Blood pressure which is acceptable.
7. Conscious level required.
8. Adequacy of pain relief: Be ready to accept that a patient is in pain and do not withhold analgesia where it is needed. It is a Royal College recommendation that there should be an acute pain service whereby all patients with either an epidural or patient-controlled analgesia (PCA) are seen every day by an anaesthetist, who may also be contacted at any time for advice. No patient with a PCA or an epidural may receive night sedation, or opiate medication by any other route. Some authorities insist on High-Dependency Unit (HDU) care for patients who have received spinal opiates. It is usual to prescribe a non-steroidal anti-inflammatory drug in conjunction with these techniques. Analgesia will otherwise be administered by the nursing staff in accordance with the anaesthetist's instructions. If it is necessary to prescribe additional analgesia, consider why it has become necessary - has something changed or gone wrong - bleeding into a joint, perforation of a viscus, etc., before writing up a stronger preparation.

Never prescribe a NSAID in renal impairment, dehydration, asthma, peptic ulceration, or risk of bleeding.

Never sedate a chronic bronchitic, especially of the CO_2 retaining type; use opiates with caution in these people.

9. Dermatomal level of regional block to be maintained if a regional technique has been used for postoperative pain relief.
10. IV access and fluids: A diuretic must UNDER NO CIRCUMSTANCES be administered without knowledge of the fluid balance and clinical state of hydration, and preferably with the knowledge

of the central venous pressure. The correct treatment of oliguria in the first instance is a fluid challenge of 3.5 ml/kg body weight of 4.5% Human Albumin Solution (HAS), or equivalent colloid, e.g. Haemaccel; See "Fluid and replacement" in the Physiology section.

11. Postoperative drugs.
12. Operation site review.
13. Other; CVP, urine output, temperature.

DAY CASE UNIT DISCHARGE CRITERIA

1. Adequate ventilation established.
2. Patient is awake and lucid.
3. Observed stability of blood pressure and heart rate and rhythm.
4. Swallow and cough reflexes restored.
5. Walking without fainting.
6. No nausea or vomiting.
7. Patient has passed urine.
8. Patient has taken fluids.
9. Operation site reviewed.
10. Postoperative instructions given, verbally and in writing, and understood by patient and carer.
11. Postoperative therapy provided.
12. GP letter sent.
13. GP phoned if indicated.
14. Follow-up arrangements made.
15. Supervision confirmed.
16. Audit form completed.

DAY CASE DISCHARGE INSTRUCTIONS

1. Instructions about observations given to carer.
2. Patient to be accompanied by an adult of "suitably robust proportions", responsible for care for next 24 hours.
3. Analgesia and postoperative instructions provided in written form with contact phone numbers in case of difficulty.
4. Warning given, pre- and postoperatively, in verbal and written form, against driving, operating machinery, cooking, childminding, and against the ingestion of alcohol or sedative drugs other than those prescribed, for a minimum of 24 hours.

POSTOPERATIVE PYREXIA

This can be due to four common causes, which may be neatly summarised as follows:

2 days:	WIND:	Chest infection.
4 days:	WATER:	Urinary tract infection.
6 days:	WOUND:	Abscess.
8 days:	WALK:	Deep vein thrombosis.

Physiology

HAEMODYNAMIC VARIABLES

Variable	Abbreviation	Formula	Normal Value
Cardiac output	CO	SV x HR	5 L/min
Cardiac index	CI	$\dfrac{CO}{BSA}$	3.2 L/min/m^2
Stroke volume	SV	$\dfrac{CO \times 1,000}{HR}$	80 ml
Stroke index	SI	$\dfrac{SV}{BSA}$	50 ml/m^2
Systemic vascular resistance	SVR	$\dfrac{MAP - CVP}{CO}$ x 80	1,000 - 1,200 dyne- sec/cm^2
Pulmonary vascular resistance	PVR	$\dfrac{PAP - LAP}{CO}$	60 -120 dyne- sec/cm^2
Ejection fraction	EF	$\dfrac{ESV - EDV}{EDV}$	> 0.6

PRESSURES: NORMAL VALUES

Right atrial pressure	1 - 7 mmHg (2 - 10 cmH20)
RV systolic	15 - 25 mmHg
RV diastolic	0 - 8 mmHg
PA systolic	15 - 25 mmHg
PA diastolic	8 - 15 mmHg
Pulmonary artery pressure	10 - 20 mmHg
Pulmonary capillary wedge pressure (PCWP)	6 - 15 mmHg

THE ARTERIAL PRESSURE SIGNAL

At least four things can be learnt from the arterial pressure signal.

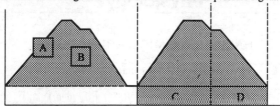

A: Rate of pressure increase is proportional to myocardial contractility.
B: Area under the curve of pulse pressure is proportional to stroke volume.
C: Systolic pressure x time is proportional to myocardial work and O_2 consumption.
D: Diastolic pressure x time is proportional to myocardial perfusion.

ARTERIO-VENOUS OXYGEN DIFFERENCE AND MIXED VENOUS OXYGEN

Taking simultaneous arterial and mixed venous (the latter from the tip of a pulmonary artery catheter) samples allows for derivation of the arterio-venous oxygen difference. The Fick equation permits calculation of $\dot{V}O_2$, Oxygen consumption.

$$\dot{V}O_2$$

Fick : $\dot{Q} = (CaO_2 - CvO_2)$
Reverse Fick: $\dot{V}O_2 = CO \times (CaO_2 - C\bar{v}O_2) \times 10$
For CaO_2 and CvO_2:
O_2 content $= (1.39 \times Hb \times Sat/100) + 0.02\ PO_2$
The $\dot{V}O_2$ can then be assessed in the light of the cardiac output at that time. Shoemaker (*Intensive Care Med* (1987) **13**:230-243) suggests that the critically ill patient requires a $\dot{V}O_2$ 30% greater than normal (N = 100 - 180 ml/min/m²). Many people now regard this, and the other Shoemaker goals, as more of a physiological test than a set of achievable targets.

MIXED VENOUS OXYGEN (SvO$_2$)

Mixed venous oxygen saturation is the percentage of mixed venous blood which is oxygenated, and may be measured photometrically at the tip of a PA catheter.

S$\bar{v}$O$_2$ is decreased with:
1. Anaemia.
2. Low cardiac output.
3. Arterial oxygen desaturation.
4. Increased oxygen consumption.

S$\bar{v}$O$_2$ is increased with:
1. Sepsis with peripheral shunting.
2. Cyanide toxicity.
3. Hypothermia.
4. A wedged PA catheter.

(From TE Oh, *Intensive Care Manual*, 3rd Ed)

VENOUS PULSE

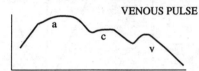

a = atrial systole. A cannon wave is a massive a-wave seen in complete heart block.
c = bulging of tricuspid valve in isovolumetric ventricular systole. Increased in tricuspid incompetence.
v = atrial filling.

LUNG VOLUMES, CAPACITIES AND LOOPS

A capacity consists of two or more volumes. Figures shown are for an adult.

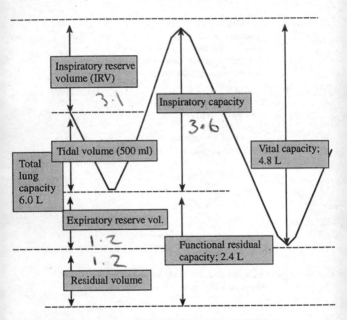

CLOSING CAPACITY = CLOSING VOLUME + RESIDUAL VOLUME: This rises with age and represents the volume of the lungs at which small airways start to close. Functional residual capacity is reduced by 20% in anaesthesia due to diaphragmatic shift, decreased ribcage dimensions and positive pressure ventilation. If FRC falls below CC, areas will be perfused but not ventilated. This explains at least part of the V/Q mismatch seen in anaesthesia and is one reason for the use of inspired fractions of oxygen of at least 0.30.

MAXIMUM BREATHING CAPACITY = maximum frequency x vital capacity (VC), sampled over 15 seconds; normal value is greater than 60 l/min; less than 25 l/min represents severe respiratory incapacity.

FVC reduction implies restrictive disease; normal is 60 ml/kg. If less than 15 ml/kg, the patient is unable to cough.
FEV1/FVC ratio reduction implies obstructive disease.

PRESSURE- AND FLOW-VOLUME LOOPS

PRESSURE-VOLUME LOOPS
These are about: Compliance = $\dfrac{\text{Volume}}{\text{Pressure}}$

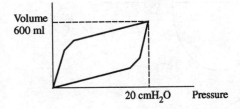

This is an example of hysteresis. In addition to quantification of disease (restrictive airways disease), it is used to represent graphically the efficiency or inefficiency of ventilation - for example, when more pressure produces no more volume. It may also demonstrate the secondary displacement of an endobronchial tube.

Compliance x resistance = the time constant, of a particular lung unit. Differing time constants within a lung represent disease and will cause pendelluft, with inefficiency of gas movement. Compliance may decrease at high frequency in this case, and dynamic, rather than static, compliance becomes a more meaningful measurement.

FLOW-VOLUME LOOPS
These are about: Resistance = $\dfrac{\text{Pressure}}{\text{Flow}}$

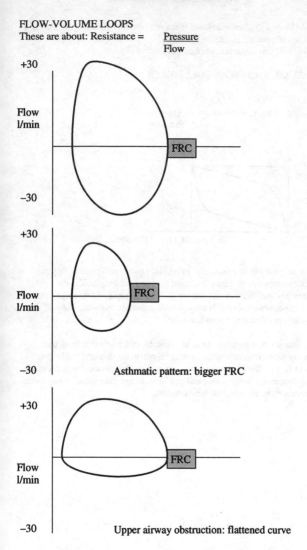

Asthmatic pattern: bigger FRC

Upper airway obstruction: flattened curve

SINGLE BREATH NITROGEN TEST

This is a modification of Fowler's method; the patient takes a slow expiration after a single breath of 100% O_2, and the nitrogen concentration in the expiration is measured. A perpendicular drawn through phase II locates $V_{D, anat}$. The slope of phase III (the alveolar plateau) defines evenness of ventilation distribution. The start of phase IV defines closing capacity.

NITROGEN (%)

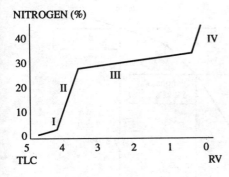

THE OXYHAEMOGLOBIN DISSOCIATION CURVE (ODC)

This relates the percentage of haemoglobin in the blood which has oxygen bound to it, to the local partial pressure of oxygen. It is best drawn through a series of known points; I have chosen the P_{50}, the P_{90} and venous blood.

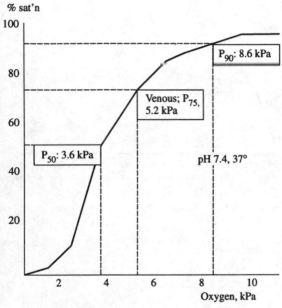

1. Hb rapidly takes on O_2 when in the pulmonary capillary;
2. Hb retains O_2 until it reaches regions of relative hypoxia.
3. Hb is 50% saturated (P_{50}) at a partial pressure of 3.6 kPa, and 90% saturated (P_{90}) at 8.6 kPa.
4. The Bohr Effect is shifting of the ODC to the right, which means that binding will be inhibited and unloading of O_2 facilitated. This is caused by: $\uparrow CO_2$, $\uparrow$ Temperature, $\uparrow [H^+]$ and $\uparrow$ 2,3 DPG.

PHYSICS AND EQUATIONS

These are the commonly-used equations, listed here for reference. A very few notes of explanation are given to explain the relevance of an equation to anaesthetic practice.

Ideal gas equation: $PV = RT$
Where P is pressure, V volume, T temperature, and R a constant. At the same temperature, P and V are inversely related; increasing pressure will reduce volume.

Dead space: $V_{D,Phys} = V_{D,Anat} + V_{D,Alv.}$
Total dead space ($V_{D,Phys}$) is made up of alveolar dead space (non-ventilated alveoli) and anatomical dead space (conducting airways). Alveolar dead space increases in disease while anatomical dead space increases with age.

Bohr equation: $V_{D,Phys} = V_T \times \dfrac{P_ACO_2 - P_ECO_2}{P_ACO_2}$
The Bohr equation assumes no CO_2 in inspired gas. The normal physiological (total) dead space, as a proportion of tidal volume, (V_D/V_T) = 0.3

To measure $V_{D,Anat}$: Fowler's method; corresponds to vertical line through phase II of the single breath nitrogen washout. Normal = 150 ml.

Alveolar ventilation equation: $V_A = \dfrac{VCO_2 \times K}{P_ACO_2}$
Where K – 0.863, if V_A is body temperature, ambient pressure, and saturated with water vapour (BTPS), and VCO_2 is standard (0°C) temperature and pressure (760 mmHg) and dry (STPD). Essentially, alveolar ventilation is proportional to CO_2 production and inversely proportional to alveolar CO_2.

This is not the same as what follows (although it is a common mistake to confuse the two):

Alveolar gas equation: $P_AO_2 \alpha$ $\quad PiO_2 - \dfrac{P_ACO_2}{R}$

The alveolar partial pressure of oxygen is dependant on the inspired fraction and on the amount of CO_2 which is, effectively, displacing the oxygen. This explains the advantage of pre-oxygenation, and explains why desaturation occurs rapidly after apnoea as the CO2 accumulates in the alveoli unless preoxygenation has been used. It also relates to altitude, and explains the mild hyperventilation seen at altitude - reduction in CO_2 allows more space for oxygen. The equation as written above assumes no CO_2 in inspired gas.

Venous admixture: this is venous blood entering the systemic arterial circulation. Venous admixture is due to frank shunt + the effects of low $\dot{V}/\dot{Q}$. Note that while $\dot{V}/\dot{Q}$ affects O_2 and CO_2, shunt only really affects oxygenation.

Shunt equation: $\quad \dfrac{Qs}{Qt} = \dfrac{Cc'O_2 - CaO_2}{Cc'O_2 - C\bar{v}O_2}$

Normal = 5 ml/100 ml.

Diffusing capacity:
The amount of gas transferred across a membrane is proportional to:
- Area
- Difference in partial pressures
- Constant
- 1/thickness

Diffusing capacity may be measured by the single breath carbon monoxide (CO) technique, where the disappearance of a single breath of CO is measured over a 10 second breath hold. Helium dilution is used to measure total lung volume at the same time.

$$D_L = \frac{VCO}{P_ACO} \quad \text{(Normal 25 ml/min/mmHg)}$$

Oxygen flux = cardiac output x oxygen content.
Oxygen content = (1.39 x Hb x Sat/100) + 0.02 PO_2

Henderson-Hasselbalch:

$$pH = pKa + \frac{\log (HCO_3^-)}{0.03 \, PCO_2}$$

This is used to calculate blood pH, which falls (blood becomes more acid) if the bicarbonate falls or the CO_2 rises.

Laplace's law: $P = \dfrac{4T}{r}$ *(Alveolus $\frac{2T}{r}$ Only one surface involved)*

Where P is the pressure in a bubble, T is the surface tension and r the radius. A small bubble (or alveolus) will collapse into a large one because it will have a larger pressure within it, due to the action of T in the walls of the alveolus. This does not happen, of course, because of the action of surfactant, which reduces the surface tension.

Pouseille's law: $Q = \dfrac{P\pi r^4}{8\mu l}$

Where Q is flow through a tube, P is the pressure difference between the ends, μ is the viscosity of the fluid and l the length of the tube. Laminar flow applies. The point is that flow through a tube, vessel or cannula is determined by the driving pressure, the viscosity and the length in a simple manner but is governed by the radius of the tube to the fourth power. So, doubling the radius of a cannula increases flow 16 times.

Fanning equation: $Q = \dfrac{P\pi^2 r^5}{fr}$

This is analogous to Pouseille's law but describes turbulent, not laminar, flow.

Reynolds number: $Re = \dfrac{2rvd}{\eta}$

This describes the possibility of turbulent flow, where r is radius, v velocity and d density, with η viscosity as before. If the number exceeds 2000, turbulent flow is likely.

The Bernouli effect is that gas passes faster through a constriction, gaining kinetic energy, but losing potential energy and so dropping pressure. If used to entrain a second gas, this is the Venturi effect. The Coanda effect is that a substance flowing in a tube is attracted to the walls. This is the basis of some ventilators.

OTHER RESPIRATORY GAS CURVES

THE SHUNT DIAGRAM

This is used to demonstrate the effect of different degrees of shunt on arterial oxygenation, in the presence of increased inspired fraction of oxygen (FiO_2). Essentially, if no shunt is present, PaO_2 will increase linearly with FiO_2. However if a large shunt is present, increasing the FiO_2 will not improve oxygenation.

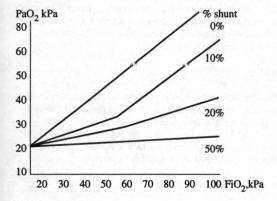

THE O₂ - CO₂ DIAGRAM

Alveolar CO_2 and alveolar O_2 cannot alter independantly one of the other; they are related. This diagram is used to display all the possible combinations of alveolar CO_2 and O_2 that can exist. A is the arterial combination, with a PO_2 of about 13 kPa and PCO_2 5.2 kPa. I is the inspired combination, with atmospheric oxygen and no carbon dioxide. V is the mixed venous combination. These points are joined by a line, movement along which is governed by alterations in V/Q, as shown.

PCO₂ (kPa)

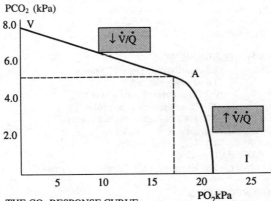

PO₂kPa

THE CO₂ RESPONSE CURVE

This relates ventilation, V, to arterial CO_2 This is one of the few relationships which is truly linear, and is displaced to the right (requiring a higher CO2 for the same ventilation) by general anaesthesia and sedation.

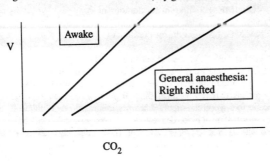

FLUIDS AND REPLACEMENT

TO CALCULATE NORMAL BLOOD VOLUME
ADULT: 7% Body Weight (Body water = 42 Litres in 70 kg man) or,
         70 ml/kg
CHILD: 80 ml/kg
NEONATE: 90 ml/kg

DAILY WATER REQUIREMENT
0-10th kg body weight:	100 ml/kg/day:
10th-20th kg body weight:	add 50 ml/kg/day:
>20th kg body weight:	add 20 ml/kg/day.

NUTRITIONAL REQUIREMENT
POTASSIUM: 1.5 mmol/kg/day (1g = 13.5 mmol)
SODIUM: 1.0 mmol/kg/day
ENERGY: in kCal = water requirement in ml
              25 - 35 non-protein kCal/kg/day
NITROGEN: 0.2 - 0.4 g N_2/kg/day (monitor urea)
MAGNESIUM: 1 mmol/g N_2
PHOSPHORUS: 0.5 - 0.75 mmol/kg/day
WATER SOLUBLE VITAMINS
TRACE ELEMENTS: Zn^+ 100 μmol, Cu^{++} 20 pmol, Mn 5 μmol, Se 0.4 μmol.
ESSENTIAL FATTY ACIDS.
Maximal rate of glucose infusion = 6.0 mg/kg/min

INTRAOPERATIVE FLUID REQUIREMENT
Add 1 + 2 + 3 + 4 = total requirement
1. INITIAL VOLUME: 1.5 ml/kg/hr for duration of
period of starvation;
2. MAINTENANCE: 1.5 ml/kg/hr for duration of
operation;
3. INSENSITIVE LOSS: E.g. opened peritoneum, 1L.
4. BLOOD LOSS: Transfuse if loss is >20% blood volume. However this
needs to be interpreted in the light of the starting haemoglobin. It has been
traditional for patients to have a haemoglobin >10 g/dl for elective surgery. This
is due to concerns for myocardial supply. The myocardium extracts 12 ml/dl of
oxygen from every 100 ml of blood delivered to the coronary circulation. The
CaO_2 of blood with a Hb of 10 g/dl is 14.5 ml/dl. This comfortably exceeds the
maximum extraction from the myocardial supply.

BURNS FLUIDS
There are a number of ways of calculating the requirement for burns fluids.
One of the best known is the Muir & Barclay formula, which covers
colloid, crystalloid and blood.
COLLOID:
(Body weight x % Body Surface Burn, BSB)/2 = ml to be transfused per
block; blocks occupy 4,4,4,6,6,12 hours post injury.
CRYSTALLOID: metabolic requirement as 5% Dextrose
1.5 x BW = ml/hr
BLOOD: 50 ml/1% BSB

STATIC PLASMA DEFICIT:
This allows calculation of how the resuscitation of a burns victim is
proceding. Take calculated blood volume (BV):

$$\text{Deficit (ml)} = BV - \frac{(BV \times \text{normal Hct})}{\text{observed Hct}}$$

CHEMISTRY AND CORRECTION

THE TENDENCY TO TETANY:

This is proportional to

$$\frac{[HCO_3^-] \times [HPO_4^-]}{[Ca^{++}] \times [Mg^{++}] \times [H^+]}$$

Such that the risk is enhanced by high bicarbonate and a low hydrogen ion concentration (in other words, by alkalosis) and by a low calcium ion concentration.

ANION GAP:

This is a measure of the presence of acid moeities. It is calculated:
$([Na+]+[K+]) - ([Cl-]+[HCO3^-])$; normal = 10-15 mmol/l

The anion gap is increased by:

- Increased serum lactate - but lactate can be directly measured now, so the anion gap has become a less frequently used measurement.
- Ketoacidosis.
- Increased foreign anions, salicylates for example.
- Low Ca^{++}, Mg^{++}, K^+.

The anion gap is decreased by:

- Hypoalbuminaemia.
- Increased plasma cations.

CALCULATION OF OSMOLARITY

= $2[Na^+ + K^+]$ + [Urea] + [Glucose]; normal = 285-295 mOsm/l.
Direct measurement by depression of freezing point indicates osmolality. Calculation indicates osmolarity. In reality, there is little difference between osmolarity and osmolality other than when there is extreme hyperlipidaemia or hyperproteinaemia. Comparison of plasma and urine must be done in terms of osmolality of both, in other words, by direct measurement.

CORRECTION OF ACIDOSIS

Base deficit (ecf) x kg body weight /3, given as ml of 8.4% Bicarbonate (1 ml = 1 mmol)
Usually, half of this is given and a repeat measurement taken. Chemical correction of acidosis is only used if the acidosis is extreme and if respiratory correction has been unsuccessful.

BLOOD COAGULATION PATHWAYS.

Primary haemostasis depends solely on platelet function. The coagulation proteins form Fibrin which stabilises the platelet clot.

The intrinsic pathway is so-called because all components circulate in plasma
$\Downarrow$ = action; $\rightarrow$ = conformational change

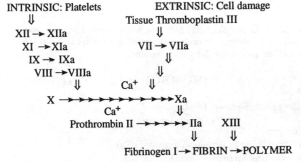

TESTS OF COAGULATION

- Platelet count: >150000/mm³
- Fibrinogen: >150 mg/100 ml
- Platelet function: Bleeding time < 10 min
- Intrinsic (heparin): KCCT < 38 sec
- Extrinsic (warfarin): PT < 16 sec. This may also be given as the International Normalised Ratio (INR) to a control using a standard thromboplastin. The ratio required depends on the condition, e.g. 2 for prophylaxis against emboli in atrial fibrillation, and 3 where a prosthetic valve is to be protected.

WARFARIN: This is a vitamin K antagonist; causing false synthesis of γ-carboxyglutamic acid residues at factors as below:

Factor:	VII	IX	X	II
Half life	2 h	17 h	40 h	60 h

Dose of warfarin: 10 mg od, until adequate INR is achieved, then maintenance with ¼ total initial dose. Reversal is possible with Vitamin K 10 mg and fresh frozen plasma if urgent.

HEPARIN: This is an antithrombin III cofactor; 100 u = 1 mg. Initial dose 5000 u, then 1000 u/hr. Heparin 4 mg/kg is used during coronary artery bypass grafting. Reversal is by Protamine 1 mg/100 u heparin. Protamine must be given with caution and slowly as a reversal dose of protamine for 4 mg/kg of heparin will consist of up to 25 ml of the standard 1% solution. Protamine causes a drop in systemic vascular resistance and an increase in pulmonary vascular resistance, and these effects are enhanced in the presence of high inspired oxygen fractions.

LOW MOLECULAR WEIGHT HEPARIN: Fractionated heparin, once daily dose, more effective in orthopaedic practice. Need factor X assay to monitor effect. Less reversible with protamine.

THROMBOLYSIS

Vascular endothelium → Prostacyclin
$\quad\quad\quad\quad\quad\quad\quad\quad$ = platelet inhibitor
Plasminogen
$\quad\downarrow\quad\Leftarrow$ Tissue Plasminogen Activator (tPa)
$\quad\downarrow\quad\Leftarrow$ Kallikrein $\quad\quad\quad$ }
$\quad\downarrow\quad\Leftarrow$ XIIa $\quad\quad\quad\quad\quad$ } both from intrinsic pathway
Plasmin $\Rightarrow$ Cleavage of Fibrin and Fibrinogen

$$\boxed{\text{FDP}}$$

TESTS:
- Fibrin degradation products; normal <10mg/l.
- D-dimer: FDP portion released only in fibrinolysis; Normal <500 ng/ml.

$$CL_H = Q \times \frac{(Cl_I \times f)}{Q + (Cl_I \times f)}$$

$$\text{Required oral dose} = \frac{Cp \times I \times Cl}{f}$$

I - dose interval
f - bioavailability

Pharmacology and statistics

PHARMACOKINETIC EQUATIONS

Pharmacokinetics is the study of what the *body* does to a *drug*, in contrast to pharmacodynamics, which is the study of what a *drug* does to the *body*. Kinetics allow for the prediction of action of drugs in normality and in altered states of metabolism.

SINGLE COMPARTMENT MODELS
Where the drug is resident in, and eliminated from, a single space.
FIRST ORDER KINETICS; Rate of elimination is proportional to amount of drug present.

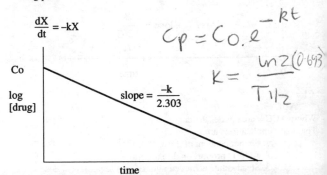

$$\frac{dX}{dt} = -kX$$

$$Cp = Co.e^{-kt}$$

$$K = \frac{\ln 2 \, (0.693)}{T_{1/2}}$$

Co

log [drug]

$$slope = \frac{-k}{2.303}$$

time

VOLUME OF DISTRIBUTION $\quad Vd = \dfrac{Xo}{Co}$ $\qquad Cl = V.k$

Where Xo is drug quantity at time O, and Co is concentration at time O.

HALF LIFE $\quad t\frac{1}{2} = \dfrac{0.693 \, Vd}{Cl}$

> independent of Xo
> dependent on volume of distribution, Vd, and clearance, Cl.

$$\text{load dose} = Cp \times Vd.$$

$$AUC = \frac{Co}{k}$$

$$\text{infusion rate} = Cp \times Cl$$

$$Cl = \frac{dose}{AUC}$$

101

TWO-COMPARTMENT MODEL

This is where the drug in question is resident in, and moves between, two spaces in the body and is eliminated from one or the other. Thiopentone is an example of this, where the rapid offset of action is due to redistribution from the plasma (the first compartment) to lipid-rich tissue, the second compartment.

α = rate constant of distribution phase
β = rate constant of elimination phase
A and B = intercepts

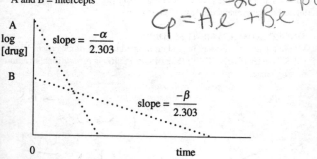

$$C_p = Ae^{-\alpha t} + Be^{-\beta t}$$

$$Cl = \frac{X_o}{AUC}$$

Where AUC = area under the curve.

The major implications are:

1. t½ independent of dose.
2. AUC is proportional to dose.
3. Steady state achieved after t½ x 4 regardless of dose.
4. Loading dose = desired plasma level x Vd
5. Infusion rate = [steady state] x Cl
6. A drug will accumulate if the dose interval, T < 1.4 x t½.

NON-LINEAR PHARMACOKINETICS

Some drugs behave as if rate-limited by the capacity of their elimination system.These include alcohol, phenytoin and salicylates.The Michaelis-Menton Equation describes saturable enzyme kinetics but can be applied to the mathematical modelling of non-linear kinetics:

$$\frac{-dC}{dt} = \frac{VmC}{Km+C}$$

where
Vm = apparent maximum rate of process
Km = [drug] at half maximum rate
C = [drug]

The implications of this are:

1. If C is far below Km, first-order kinetics apply.

2. If C is far above Km, the decline in concentration proceeds at a fixed rate; this is zero-order kinetics.

3. The time required to eliminate 50% of dose increases with increased dose: no constant t½.

4. AUC is proportional to square of the dose; small increase in dose can cause huge increase in amount of drug in body, once the elimination process is saturated.

5. More than one drug may use the same route of elimination in which case competition occurs.

PHARMACODYNAMICS

This is the study of what the *drug* does to the *body*. In contrast to pharmacokinetics, this is very difficult to model mathematically as the mechanism of action of drugs is complex, systems may become saturated, and plasma values of a drug may bear little resemblance to the concentration at the site of action; psychotropic drugs are examples. A drug may have complicated effects which outlast the presence of the agent itself; steroids are an example of this. Finally, some agents do observe a close relationship between amount present and observed effect; these are mostly receptor-based in their action and include remifentanil at the μ receptor, inotropes on α and β receptors, and nitroprusside in its action on smooth muscle.

The log dose-response curve is the typical diagram used to describe pharmaco dynamic relationships. The use of logarithms allows for curved relationships to become linear, interactions to be more easily spotted and for easier calculation of effective doses.

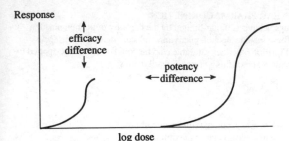

For example, fentanyl is more potent than alfentanil, so the log dose-response curves will be the same shape (that is, both reaching 100% response) but they will be separated on the x-axis. Dihydrocodeine is not as efficacious as fentanyl, so the log dose-response curves for these two drugs will not be the same shape, the curve for dihydrocodeine never reaching the same height on the y-axis as fentanyl.

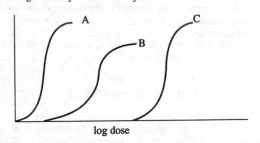

A: Drug with high affinity and high intrinsic activity: true agonist: fentanyl.
B: Drug with high affinity but less intrinsic activity: Partial agonist; never reaches 100% response: Buprenorphine.
C: Agonist in presence of antagonist; agonist will reach 100% response even in the presence of the antagonist, as long as the dose of agonist is great enough; fentanyl and naloxone.

Schild equation :- Dose ratio - 1 = Ka [A]
Ka - antagonist affinity constant
PA₂ - -ve log of molar dose antagonist → dose ratio of 2.

THE IDEALS

THE IDEAL INDUCTION AGENT

PHYSICAL:
Water soluble
Stable in solution
No adsorption onto plastic
Cheap to synthesise
Compatible with other drugs
PHARMACOKINETIC:
Sleep in one arm-brain circulation time
Short and predictable duration of action
Not cumulative
Inactivation by metabolism to inactive metabolites
PHARMACODYNAMIC:
No pain on injection
No cardiovascular or respiratory effects
Analgesic
No histamine release
No increase in muscle tone or excitatory movements
No interactions
No effects on the gravid uterus
Safe if extravasated or given intra-arterially

TOTAL INTRAVENOUS ANAESTHESIA (TIVA)

This is the technique of using an induction agent both for induction of anaesthesia and as a continuous infusion to maintain anaesthesia. It avoids the use of volatile agents. This may be useful in avoiding nausea, vomiting, enhancement of neuromuscular blockade, atmospheric pollution and the risk of Malignant Hyperpyrexia. There is a risk of awareness if disconnection occurs; also, Minimum Infusion Rate (which is analogous to MAC) is poorly defined for most agents.

These are some examples:

1. PROPOFOL 50 ml, mixed with ALFENTANIL 1.5 mg; 1.0 mg/kg propofol for induction, followed by 10 mg/kg/hr, then 8 mg/kg/hr then 6 mg/kg/hr. This may be used for spontaneously breathing or paralysed and ventilated patients.

2. KETAMINE 200 mg, MIDAZOLAM 5 mg, VECURONIUM 12 mg, made up to 50 ml with saline. Induction: Ketamine 1.0 mg/kg with midazolam 0.07 mg/kg; thereafter body weight/2 in ml/hr of the mixture. Intermittent positive pressure ventilation is provided with O_2 in air.

3. KETAMINE 200 mg, MIDAZOLAM 5 mg, ALFENTANIL 1 mg all in 50 ml saline. Induction: Ketamine 2 mg/kg with midazolam 0.07 mg/kg; thereafter body weight/2 in ml/hr of the mixture for maintenance, with spontaneous respiration of O_2 in air, which may be augmented with isoflurane, although this would then cease to be true TIVA.

ADMINISTRATION OF TIVA

This is by syringe driver although the earliest examples used simple drip sets. The Graseby model 3400 allows calculation of rate based on body weight.

CLAN is closed loop anaesthesia and involves use of the auditory evoked response to adjust the amount of TIVA administered.

THE IDEAL INHALATIONAL AGENT

PHYSICAL:
Stable in light, heat, metal, soda-lime
No preservatives
Long shelf life
Not flammable or explosive in air, N_2O or oxygen
Non irritant
Atmospherically friendly
Cheap to synthesise
PHARMACOKINETIC:
High oil:gas coefficient, so low MAC
Low blood:gas coefficient, so fast effects
Not metabolised
PHARMACODYNAMIC:
Non toxic, even in chronic, low dose
No cardiovascular or respiratory effects
Analgesic
Readily reversible CNS effects
Not epileptogenic
No interactions
No effects on the gravid uterus

CHARACTERISTICS OF VOLATILE ANAESTHETIC AGENTS

	MAC	BP	SVP	B:G	O:G	Mw
Halothane	0.7	50	33%	2.3	224	197
Enflurane	1.7	56	24%	1.8	98.5	184
Isoflurane	1.17	49	33%	1.4	99	184
Sevoflurane	1.9	55	24%	0.6	53	200
Desflurane	6.0	23	88%	0.4	20	168

MAC: Minimum Alveolar Concentration, which is the amount of the agent delivered in oxygen at room temperature at sea level which will keep 50% of unpremedicated experimental animals still at skin incision.
It is reduced by:

> 1. Age (10% per decade)
> 2. Premedication
> 3. Opioids
> 4. Hypovolaemia.
> 5. Reduced temperature
> 6. Other drugs; for example, clonidine, dexmedetomidine
> 7. Disease; hypothyroidism

BP: Boiling point, in °C.
SVP: The pressure exerted by the vapour phase above the liquid phase at equilibrium, in other words when as many molecules are leaving the liquid as returning. This depends on the agent and its temperature and is independant of atmospheric pressure. It defines the calibration of the vaporiser.
B:G: Blood:gas partition coefficient: the less soluble the agent, the more rapid the onset and offset of action
O:G: Oil:gas partition coefficient: this bears a linear inverse relationship to MAC and is therefore an indicator of potency.
MW: Molecular weight, in Daltons.

CALCULATION OF INFUSION RATES

1% = 10 mg in 1 ml;
1:10,000 = 1 gram in 10,000 ml

1 ml = 15 normal drops = 60 microdrops
∴1 ml/hour = 1 microdrop/minute
1 L over 12 hr = 83 ml/hr = 20 drops per minute
1 L over 8 hr = 125 ml/hr = 30 drops per minute
1 L over 6 hr = 166 ml/hr = 40 drops per minute
1 L over 4 hr = 250 ml/hr = 60 drops per minute

TO CALCULATE INFUSION RATES:
$$\frac{\text{Dose you want to give (mcg/kg/min)} \times \text{Vol} \times \text{kg body wt} \times 60}{\text{Amount of drug in infusion (mcg)}}$$

TO SIMPLIFY
3 mg of drug into 50 ml
1 ml/hr = 1 mcg/min

BY BODY WEIGHT
(Body weight in kg x 3) mg of drug into 50 ml
1 ml/hr = 1 mcg/kg/min

COMMON INFUSIONS: ADULTS

DRUG	PRESENTATION	DOSE
ADRENALINE	1 mg ampoule (1:1,000)	1 - 4 mcg/min
ALFENTANIL	5 mg ampoule	0.5 - 1.0 mcg/kg/min
AMINOPHYLLINE	250 mg ampoule	0.2 - 0.9 mg/kg/hr
AMIODARONE	150 mg ampoule	5 mg/kg; loading dose
BRETYLIUM	500 mg ampoule	5 - 10 mg/kg loading dose; 1 - 2 mg/min
DOPAMINE	200 mg ampoule	1.0 - 15 mcg/kg/min
DOPEXAMINE	50 mg ampoule	0.5 - 6.0 mcg/kg/min
DOBUTAMINE	250 mg ampoule	2 - 10 mcg/kg/min
ENOXIMONE	100 mg ampoule	0.5 mg/kg loading dose; 5 - 20 mcg/kg/min
FENTANYL	0.5 mg ampoule	0.02 - 0.05 mcg/kg/min
GTN	50 mg ampoule	5 - 200 mcg/min
ISOPRENALINE	1 mg ampoule	1.0 - 10 mcg/min
LIGNOCAINE	1 gram ampoule	100 mg loading dose, 2 - 4 mg/min
MAGNESIUM SULPHATE	5 g ampoule	1-2 g loading dose, 2-2.5 g/h
NITROPRUSSIDE	50 mg ampoule	up to 1.5 mcg/kg/min
NORADRENALINE	2 or 4 mg ampoule	4.0 - 12 mcg/min
TRIMETAPHAN	500 mg ampoule	3 - 4 mg/min

RELAXANTS

Neuromuscular blockade is usually maintained by the use of non-depolarising agents, although some practitioners still favour the suxamethonium drip technique. Non-depolarisers can be given by intermittent bolus or by infusion.

VECURONIUM 10 mg in 5 ml of buffered freeze-dried bromide as powder for reconstitution. Contains mannitol.	Dose (mcg/kg)	Dose (mg for a 70 kg patient)	Volume of dose for 70 kg (ml)
Intubation	100	7	3.5
Maintenance (Bolus)	50	3.5	1.7
Maintenance (Infusion)/hour	80	5.5	2.5
ATRACURIUM 50 mg in 5 ml yellow coloured solution of the besylate; stored at 2 - 8°Celsius	Dose (mcg/kg)	Dose (mg for a 70 kg patient)	Volume of dose for 70 kg (ml)
Intubation	600	40	4
Maintenance (Bolus)	200	15	1.5
Maintenance (Infusion)/hour	600	40	4
MIVACURIUM 20 mg in 10 ml clear solution of the chloride.	Dose (mcg/kg)	Dose (mg for a 70 kg patient)	Volume of dose for 70 kg (ml)
Intubation	150	10	5

Maintenance (Bolus)	100	7	3.5
Maintenance (Infusion)/hour	600	40	20

INOTROPES

DRUG	Property	Typical Dose
DOPAMINE	D>β>α	2.5 mcg/kg/min
DOBUTAMINE	β1>β2>α	2 - 10 mcg/kg/min
ADRENALINE	α,β1,β2	1 - 4 mcg/min
NORADRENALINE	α>β1	4 - 12 mcg/min
DOPEXAMINE	β2>β1>D	0.5 - 6 mcg/kg/min
EPHEDRINE	α>β1>β2	30 mg incrementally
ISOPRENALINE	β1>β2	1 - 10 mcg/min
METARAMINOL	α	10 mg incrementally
PHENYLEPHRINE	α	100 - 500 mcg bolus
SALBUTAMOL	β2>β1	250mcg,-10mcg/min
XAMOTEROL	β1	200 mg od

PREVENTION OF TACHYPHYLAXIS: some advocate the use of acetylcysteine by infusion to provide metabolic substrate.

ANTIARRHYTHMICS

Antiarrhythmics control the rhythm of the cardiac contraction usually by reducing the excitability of the conducting system or of the myocardium.

THE CARDIAC ACTION POTENTIAL (AP)

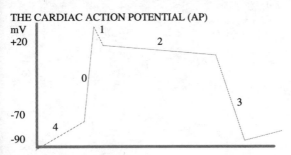

0 = Fast depolarisation, Na^+ inwards
1 = Early incomplete repolarisation
2 = Plateau, slow Ca^{++} inwards, prolonging AP
3 = Rapid repolarisation, K^+ outwards
4 = Electrical diastole, refractory period.

112

VAUGHAN-WILLIAMS CLASSIFICATION

Ia $\downarrow Na^+$ entry in phase 0; $\uparrow$repolarisation; disopyramide
 b $\downarrow Na^+$ entry in phase 0; $\downarrow$repolarisation; lignocaine, mexilitine
 c $\downarrow Na^+$ entry in phase 0; flecainidc
II β-blockade; propranolol, metoprolol.
III $\uparrow$repolarisation; bretylium, amiodarone
IV Ca ++ blockade; verapamil, nifedipine.

RECOMMENDATIONS FOR SPECIFIC ARRHYTHMIAS

VENTRICULAR ARRHYTHMIAS: lignocaine 100 mg then 2 - 4 mg/min, or mexilitine.
ATRIAL FIBRILLATION WITHOUT COMPROMISE: digoxin 1 mg divided in 24h, then 125 - 150 mcg/day; or DC shock after anticoagulation and stopping digoxin.
ATRIAL FIBRILLATION WITH COMPROMISE: DC Shock
FAST ATRIAL FIBRILLATION OF RECENT ONSET: flecainide 2 mg/kg then 1.5 mg/kg in one hour then 100 - 250 mcg/kg/hr.
WOLFF-PARKINSON-WHITE SYNDROME: amiodarone 5 mg/kg slow bolus then 200 mg/day
LOCAL ANAESTHETIC TOXICITY: bretylium 7 mg/kg then 2 mg/min infusion
SUPRAVENTRICULAR TACHYCARDIA OF RECENT ONSET: adenosine 3 mg, doubling until effect seen
SUPRAVENTRICULAR TACHYCARDIA: verapamil 5 - 10 mg slow bolus
TORSADES DES POINTES: magnesium 4 g bolus then infusion 1 g/hr, aim for 2 - 3.5 mmol/l

PAEDIATRIC DOSAGES AND CALCULATIONS

DRUGS

PREMEDICANTS:	
ATROPINE	20 mcg/kg
GLYCOPYRROLATE	40 mcg/kg
TRIMEPRAZINE	2 mg/kg
DIAZEPAM	0.1 - 0.2 mg/kg
PROMETHAZINE	0.5 - 1.0 mg/kg
MIDAZOLAM	0.5 - 0.75 mg/kg
ANTIEMETICS:	
ONDANSETRON	100 - 200 mcg/kg
METOCLOPRAMIDE	150 mcg/kg
AT THE NEUROMUSCULAR JUNCTION:	
ATRACURIUM	0.5 mg/kg
NEOSTIGMINE	50 mcg/kg
ANALGESIA:	
MORPHINE PCA	Loading: 100mcg/kg Background: 5 - 10 mcg/kg/hr Demand: 20 mcg/kg Lockout: 10 -20 minutes 4 hour limit: 400 mcg/kg
PARACETAMOL	15 mg/kg po, or 20 mg/kg pr.
CODEINE PHOSPHATE	1 mg/kg
BUPIVACAINE	Caudal to L4: 0.5 ml/kg of 0.25%, up to 2 mg/kg Caudal, to T6: 1 ml/kg of 0.25%, up to 2 mg/kg Lumbar: 0.75 ml/kg of 0.25%, up to 2 mg/kg
RESUSCITATION:	
ADRENALINE	0.1 ml/kg of 110,000
BICARBONATE	1 mmol/kg
LIGNOCAINE	1 mg/kg
DC SHOCK	1 - 2 J/kg

DEHYDRATION

Appears at loss of 5% of circulating volume = 50 ml/kg
Obvious at loss of 10% of circulating volume = 100 ml/kg
Manifest at loss of 15% of circulating volume = 150 ml/kg

DAILY FLUID REQUIREMENT

0-10th kg body weight	100 ml/kg/day
10th-20th kg body weight	add 50 ml/kg/day
>20th kg body weight	add 20 ml/kg/day.

Approximately 4 ml/kg/hr in theatre.

BLOOD REPLACEMENT

Blood volume 90 ml/kg (neonate), 80 ml/kg (child).
Transfuse 10 ml blood/kg body weight for every g/dl required
Note that paediatric cardiac index is twice that of an adult = 4.8 - 6.0
$L/min/m^2$, and that oxygen consumption, VO_2, is also twice the adult = 6.8
ml/kg/min

VENTILATION

THE NEWTON VALVE

Set times and pressures, estimate volumes.
Inspiratory time 1.0 sec
Expiratory time 1.5 sec
Peak inspiratory pressure 15 cmH$_2$O
FiO_2 0.3
Fresh gas flow 1.0 litre + (200 ml/kg) per minute

PAEDIATRIC ENDOTRACHEAL TUBE SIZES
NEONATE:
10 cm tube, 3.0 mm internal diameter.
OVER THREE MONTHS:
Internal diameter (mm) = Age/4 + 4
Length   (cm) = 12 + Age/2

THE EPIDURAL SPACE

Depth is: 1 + 0.15 x age (years), or 0.8 + 0.05 x weight (kg).
It should be located using loss of resistance to saline to avoid the risk of
venous air embolism, which can be catastrophic. A test dose with
adrenaline will not reliably detect venous placement.

MISUSE OF DRUGS REGULATIONS

SCHEDULES refer to the regulations governing the use of drugs, from the Misuse of Drugs Regulations 1985.
CLASSES refer to the harmfulness of the drugs and the penalties for misuse, from the Misuse of Drugs Act, 1971, which replaced the Dangerous Drugs Act.

SCHEDULE 1
Includes non-medicinal drugs such as cannabis and lysergide.

SCHEDULE 2
Imposes requirements for prescribing cocaine, heroin, morphine. Full dispensing record must be kept. Drugs kept in locked container.

SCHEDULE 3
Includes barbiturates and buprenorphine; subject to special prescribing requirements, but not to safe custody requirements; nor is a register required.

SCHEDULE 4
Includes the benzodiazepines. As for Schedule 3, but no special prescribing requirements.

SCHEDULE 5
Includes preparations which require only retention of invoices for two years.

CLASS A
Alfentanil, morphine, opium, heroin, methadone, pethidine, cocaine, LSD, injectable amphetamines.

CLASS B
Oral amphetamines, cannabis, codeine.

CLASS C
Amphetamine derivatives, and most benzodiazepines.

STATISTICS

DEFINITIONS

A PARAMETER is a characteristic or feature; it may be a measurement, like blood pressure, or an outcome, as whether a patient is dead or alive.

A POPULATION consists of a group which share a parameter; for example, all the males in a town, or all patients over 80 years of age.

A SAMPLE is a selection of individuals from a population who are characterised by the parameter of interest.

A MEAN is the arithmentical average, i.e. the sum of all measurements divided by the number in the group.

A MEDIAN is that measurement which lies exactly between each end of a range of values ranked in order.

A MODE is the most commonly observed value.

A NORMAL DISTRIBUTION is one where the mean, median and mode are the same.

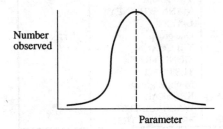

DESCRIPTIVE statistics produce means, medians and modes; measures of central tendency.

ANALYTICAL statistics are the same as inferential statistics; they assess a probability of something being the case, or of a relationship existing between two parameters, or whether two samples come from the same population.

THE NULL HYPOTHESIS is the assertion that a relationship, such as a difference, does not exist. Analytical methods start by stating the null hypothesis and setting about disproving it, i.e. proving that the relationship does exist.

PROBABILITY is expressed as a p value; it is written as a decimal but expresses a set of odds; for example, p=0.05 expresses a 1:20 chance of the null hypothesis being correct, i.e. no relationship existing. $p < 0.05$ is usually accepted for biological systems, while p<0.005 is often required for mechanical systems.

INTERVAL SCALE DATA are mathematically related real numbers and may or may not be normally distributed; e.g. BP.

RATIO DATA have all characteristics of interval scale with an implicit zero, e.g. length.

ORDINAL DATA are where an order applies; e.g. pain score.

NOMINAL DATA are yes or no; e.g. survivors or non-survivors.

PARAMETRIC TESTS should apply only to normally-distributed data.

WHICH TEST TO USE?

INTERVAL SCALE normally distributed data	ORDINAL and non-normally distributed interval scale data	NOMINAL data
Two groups UNPAIRED t-TEST	Two groups MANN-WHITNEY U-TEST	χ^2 TEST
One group PAIRED t-TEST	One group WILCOXON SIGNED-RANK TEST	
Multiple groups ONE-WAY ANOVA	Multiple groups KRUSKAL-WALLACE TEST	
TWO-WAY ANOVA	FRIEDMAN TEST	

T-TEST Produces t value and, depending upon degrees of freedom, p is then read from a table.

$$t = \frac{\overline{d}}{SE}$$

VARIANCE $= \dfrac{\Sigma(x-\bar{x})}{n-1}$

STANDARD DEVIATION $= \sqrt{\dfrac{\Sigma(x-\bar{x})}{n-1}}$

STANDARD ERROR OF THE MEAN $= SD\Big/\sqrt{n}$

ODDS RATIO is the estimate of the risk of an outcome, given some exposure or risk factor.

		Outcome YES	Outcome NO
Exposure	YES	a	b
	NO	c	d

Odds Ratio, OR $= \dfrac{ad}{bc}$

CONFIDENCE INTERVALS usually quoted as the 95% confidence intervals; this means the intervals within which 95% of values will fall. This means that if any number of samples were taken from the same population, 95% of these samples would lie within the confidence intervals. 99% confidence limits could also be quoted, but this is rarely seen.

POWER OF A TEST describes the likelihood of detecting a real difference if it exists = [(1 - type II error) x 100%]

TYPE I ERROR (α error) is a false positive. The commonest reason is multiple testing.

TYPE II ERROR (β error) is a false negative. This may be because the sample space is too small.

This applies when setting up a trial; one might say "I will accept a false positive outcome of 1:20"; this is the same as accepting a p value of p=0.05.

CORRELATION is a measure of the degree of association between two parameters.

A REGRESSION LINE is a line constructed on a graph to describe the relationship between two parameters which are approximately linearly linked.

RESEARCH AND PUBLISHING

WRITING A PROTOCOL
This precedes the setting up of a trial and is an important part of the process; it will be seen by the members of the Ethics Committee of the hospital where the study will be taking place.

TITLE Explain project and name investigations.

INTRODUCTION Need for work.

AIM One sentence.

STATEMENT OF PROBLEM Enlarges introduction.

DETAILS OF METHOD Exact procedure; possible problems and way around them.

ANALYSIS AND INTERPRETATION Include power of study and statistical methods.

APPLICATION OF FINDINGS Practical benefit.

PROPOSED SCHEDULE Start & finish, duration of each part.

FACILITIES AVAILABLE Involvement of other departments e.g. biochemistry.

FINANCE

WRITING A PAPER
It is conventional to set out a paper as follows. Always adhere to the published guidelines of the journal to which you intend submitting the paper.

ABSTRACT Why, how, findings, meanings.

KEY WORDS from MeSH headings.

INTRODUCTION What is known, what needs doing.

MATERIALS AND METHODS What I used, what I did, to whom, how. Statistical methods used.

RESULTS

DISCUSSION Implications, are conclusions valid, agreement with others, more research needed.

ACKNOWLEDGEMENTS

REFERENCES

VANCOUVER CRITERIA FOR AUTHORSHIP

This sets out what is required for an individual to be considered worthy of authorship;(a), (b) and (c) must be all be met.

(a) Conception and design of the trial, or analysis and interpretation of the data;

(b) Drafting or revising the article critically for important intellectual content;

(c) Final approval of the version to be published.

DECLARATION OF HELSINKI

This deals with the setting up of a trial and is principally intended for the protection of the participants.

1. Moral and scientific justification for study.
2. Carried out by scientifically qualified persons working under medical supervision.
3. Consideration of scientific benefit to subject risk ratio.
4. Risk of alteration to subject personality is usually unacceptable, for example by use of hallucinogenic drugs.
5. Consent of subjects.
6. Protection of subjects.

Audit and administration

AUDIT is the systematic peer review of all areas of clinical practice with the object of maintaining and improving the quality of that practice; "the systematic and critical analysis of the quality of clinical care...the associated use of resources and the resulting outcome and quality of life for the patient." (NHSME: Clinical Audit: Meeting and improving standards of Healthcare).

RESEARCH is the discipline of improving medical care by expanding the known areas of medical science, whereas audit is monitoring practice within those known areas.

PUBLICATIONS can be obtained both through audit and research. Audit rarely involves a departure from accepted clinical practice and doesn't have a control group. Hence ethics committee approval is rarely needed for audit projects.

THE AUDIT LOOP

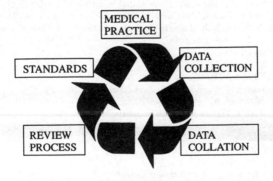

"It has long been a cornerstone of anaesthetic practice in the UK that our actions should be held up to our peers for regular review" *Graham 1992*

CONFIDENTIAL ENQUIRY INTO MATERNAL DEATHS

Beecher and Todd, 1952. This has reported every 3 years since then, and is the longest-established medical audit project. It considers maternal death up to 42 days postpartum. Since 1984 this has considered the whole UK. There is a considerable time delay between the information gathering and the publication of the report.

FINDINGS: 10† per 100,000 births (1988-90). This is unchanged from previous years. The risk of death from anaesthesia is 1.7 per million pregnancies. The total of 145 deaths in this report were attributable to the following factors;

1. Hypertensive disease   27 (18.6%)
2. Pulmonary embolus   24 (16.6%)
3. Haemorrhage   22 (15.2%)
4. Ectopic   15 (10.3%)
5. Amniotic fluid embolism 11 (7.6%)
6. Abortion   9 (6.2%)
7. Sepsis   7 (4.8%)
8. Anaesthesia   4 (2.8%)

There was also one late death due to anaesthesia. Of the 5 total, 3 involved tracheal tube problems. There were 10 cases where anaesthesia contributed to death, in which tracheal tube misplacement featured in 6. Obesity was a factor in 3 of the 4 direct deaths.

9. Ruptured uterus   2 (1.4%)

RECOMMENDATIONS:
1. Capnography should be used where general anaesthesia is administered.
2. More use of H_2 antagonists and antacids.
3. Gastric emptying should be practiced before induction of general anaesthesia.
4. Establish early big venous access.
5. Better postoperative care.
6. Development of departmental guidelines.
7. Pulse oximetry up to 48 hours in certain conditions.

CONFIDENTIAL ENQUIRY INTO PERIOPERATIVE DEATHS

1956: Association of Anaesthetists of Great Britain and Ireland: considered 1000 cases.

1987: Confidential Enquiry into Perioperative Death (CEPOD): dealt with London only.

1989: National CEPOD (NCEPOD) 1: England and Wales, sample only.

1990: NCEPOD 2. E&W, NI, Guernsey, Isle of Man, Jersey.

1993: NCEPOD 3: 010491-310392; considered death in hospital within 30 days of surgery; 12612 reports, 15% sampled. Return rate 68.9% surgical, 61.2% anaesthetic. Index cases were the most recent patient procedure. Conclusions and recommendations were laid out in different format from previous reports, but emphasised shortages of emergency theatres and ITU facilities, the fact that futile operations were carried out and that DVT was still an important and preventable cause of death. The anaesthetic recommendations were for teams, better monitoring at induction, and more use of protocols.

1995: NCEPOD 4: 010492-310393; again, death in hospital within 30 days. This report concentrated on age 6-70, and was the largest so far, with 19816 reports. Return rate was improved, at 72.4% surgical and 77.4% of anaesthetic questionnaires. General recommendations included identification of a continuing shortage of HDU and ITU facilities, advocated supervision of trainees with less than 3 years experience, and recommended early conversion to open procedure at laparoscopy when problems arise. Quality of notes and lost patient records were further concerns, and the issue of "Standard of Practice", with particular reference to anaesthesia, was raised.

Key Issues in Anaesthesia:

Standards of practice could be written for:

- Preop visiting and assessment
- Experienced staff for sick patients
- Trained non-medical staff for assistance
- Monitoring throughout
- Fully staffed and equipped recovery areas
- Pulse oximetry in recovery

Protocols could be developed for:
- DVT and PE prophylaxis
- Interhospital transfer
- Referral of sick patients to senior staff
- Essential preoperative investigations
- Retention of staff records and duty rosters
- Out of hours operating (defined as between 18:01 and 07:59 and all day at the weekend)

THE LAW AND EQUIPMENT

ELECTRICAL SAFETY
MACROSHOCK: At 5 mA there will be pain, at 50 mA paralysis, at 100 mA ventricular fibrillation (VF).
MICROSHOCK: This occurs via an intracardiac catheter, for example a central line; just 0.1 mA can cause VF.
HTM (Health Technical Memorandum) II, 1977; This deals with antistatic precautions, and these being allowed to lapse.
ELECTROMED:
CLASSES
       I earthed
       IIA no exposed metal earthed
       IIB double insulated.
TYPES   BF external surgery
       CF cardiac; lower current leakage.
DIATHERMY: What the words mean:
COAGULATION: pulsed current.
CUTTING: continuous current.
BIPOLAR: 40 Watts delivered.
MONOPOLAR: 150 - 400 Watts delivered.

SUCTION
FEATURES: Valve, gauge (anticlockwise), filter with cut-off valve to prevent contamination of central reservoir, collecting reservoir with antifoaming agent.
STANDARDS: (For anaesthetic purposes); 10 sec to generate -500 mmHg with displacement capacity of 25 l/min. Tubing needs to have low resistance and low compliance.

SCAVENGING
The threshold of smell is 33 parts per million (ppm). N_2O is a greenhouse gas, it depresses methionine synthase and causes abortion (Cohen), although this is contentious. Volatiles are HCFCs (not CFCs) and have minimal effect on the ozone layer.

CONTROL OF SUBSTANCES HAZARDOUS TO HEALTH (COSHH) 1988: It is a criminal offence not to apply this act since the lifting of Crown Immunity. It sets requirements for alternatives to mask anaesthesia, named manager with responsibility for implementation, closed system filling for vaporisers to be carried out in a fume cupboard, and minimum rates of air supply:

- Operating Theatres: $0.65 \text{ m}^3/\text{s}$
- Anaesthetic rooms: $0.15 \text{ m}^3/\text{s}$
- Prep rooms: $0.1 \text{ m}^3/\text{s}$
- Recovery: 15 air changes per hour.

It also lays down time weighted average exposure levels for volatiles, to be monitored by the use of personal samplers to be carried within the breathing area of the practitioner. These are:

- N_2O: 100 ppm (USA: 25 ppm)
- Isoflurane: 50 ppm (USA, for all volatiles, limit is 2 ppm)
- Enflurane: 20 ppm
- Halothane: 10 ppm

OTHER METHODS:
ACTIVATED CHARCOAL: Cardiff aldasorber; weighs 1 kg when new. Takes up volatiles, not N_2O.
SODA-LIME: Consists of 90% CaOH, 5% NaOH, 1% KOH and silicate (to form granules), moisture and an indicator. Takes up CO_2, produces moisture and heat. There is a risk of degradation of volatiles by dry soda-lime, to produce toxic products.
ACTIVE SCAVENGING: Consists of:
- Collecting system (30 mm connections)
- Transfer system (with pressure release valve to prevent barotrauma)
- Disposal system.

Systems should not permit pressure greater than 2 kPa at flows of 90 l/min.

STERILIZATION

This can be considered as decontamination, disinfection, and sterilization. The three are not the same.

DECONTAMINATION: This is the removal of infected matter.

DISINFECTION: This is the destruction of organisms but not spores. Methods are:

1. Pasteurisation; water, 70°c for 20 min or 80°c for 10 min; used for plastics.
2. Boiling.
3. Chlorhexidine 0.05%; used for skin.
4. Glutaraldehyde 2%; for endoscopes.
5. Sodium hypochlorite 10%; for benches and surfaces.

STERILIZATION: This kills organisms and spores. Methods are:

1. Autoclaving; pressurised steam, 130°c; for instruments and tubes. Indicator paper shows autoclaved wrapping.
2. Dry heat; 160°c; for delicate instruments.
3. Ethylene oxide; for whole machines, only available in specialist centres. It causes pulmonary oedema, so equipment must be left to elute for 10 days.
4. Gamma irradiation; for disposables.

INFECTION RISK TO STAFF

The hazards are from exposure to diseases such as TB, Hepatitis, and AIDS. The Association of Anaesthetists recommend the wearing of gloves for all procedures where the anaesthetist comes into contact with the patient. Most Trusts now insist on documentary evidence of immunisation against Hepatitis B. In the event of a needlestick injury:

1. Thoroughly clean the wound site.
2. Report incident to local manager.
3. Take blood from patient for hepatitis B (HB) status.
4. Take blood from victim for HB immune status.

ABORTION ACT 1967

Form HSA1 (green) is signed by 2 doctors, certifying that there is a risk, greater than if the pregnancy was terminated,
1. To the life of the pregnant woman.
2. To the physical or mental health of the pregnant woman.
3. To the physical or mental health of the existing child(ren).
4. That if the child were born it would suffer from such physical or mental abnormalities as to be seriously handicapped.

THE BUSINESS PLAN

This may be set out as below.
1. MISSION STATEMENT.
Specific to provision of anaesthetic services, but consistent with the Mission Statement of the Trust.
2. AIMS AND OBJECTIVES.
3. SERVICE CAPACITY
      a. Organisation and management.
      b. Staffing: Consultants, university posts, trainees, research staff, career grades, non-medical and adminstrative staff.
      c. Facilities: Theatres, ITU, pain clinics, office space, laboratory, library, teaching space, computers, accomodation.
      d. Allocation of time, notional half days (NHD). Also commitment to committee work and teaching.
4. UTILIZATION
Activity tables for previous year; Korner data.
      a. Cases, hours, and breakdown by specialty and NCEPOD categories.
      b. ITU
      c. Obstetrics
      d. Chronic Pain
      e. Acute Pain
      f. Resus and A&E activities
      g. Teaching
      h. Special interests

5. FINANCIAL RESOURCES
6. SWOT

Strengths, Weaknesses, Opportunities, Threats: PEST
                                                                  Political
                                                                  Economic
                                                                  Sociological
                                                                 Technological

7. AIMS AND OBJECTIVES

For the following year.

RISK MANAGEMENT

This is the management of an unexpected adverse event befalling a patient under anaesthetic care anywhere in the hospital. The objects are to limit damage, prevent recurrence, and protect the clinician and department from litigation.

1. Clinical director notified, Patient Care Committee informed.
2. Second clinician assumes care of patient.
3. Clinician involved completes factual account of events.
4. Location sealed for investigation by investigator.
5. Spokesman appointed for liaison with family of patient; family informed.
6. All documentation photocopied.
7. Medical defence organisations involved.
8. Systematic investigation, if appropriate, to determine causation, and prevent repetition.

REPORTING ADVERSE REACTIONS

Adverse reactions should be reported to The Committee on Safety of Medicines, London SW8 5BR using the Yellow Card scheme. With newer drugs, (denoted with an inverted triangle in data sheets and in the British National Formulary) all reactions should be reported. With established drugs, serious suspected reactions should be notified.

ADROIT = Adverse Reactions On-Line Reporting system.

Phone numbers:

CSM London: 0171 627 3291

CSM Mersey: 0151 236 4620 x 2126

CSM Wales: 01222 744181

CSM Northern: 0191 232 1525

(See also Management of Allergic Reactions, in Resuscitation and Critical Incident Management Section).

Intensive care

THE ITU ADMISSION

The use of this scheme will avoid the omission of any detail in the admission of a patient to the Intensive Care Unit or in the subsequent management.

ADMISSION
Emergency or elective admission/age/gender
Past medical history and drug history/allergy/addiction; any drugs up to and including morning of operation?

If admission is the result of trauma:
Mechanism and time of injury/velocity/restrained?
Vital signs at scene/scores/others injured

Anaesthetic time/operation/complications.
Blood loss/fluid replacement/urine output peroperatively.
Lines in situ/urinary catheter.
Airway/ventilation figures/FiO$_2$.

Specific requirements: Inotropes/antibiotics/DVT prophylaxis/feeding; eventual disposal.

EXAMINATION AND REVIEW
Top of sheet: Date / Day number / Temperature
- CNS: Glasgow coma scale/AVPU/localising signs.
- CVS: BP/heart rate/heart sounds/central pressures/output studies/SpO$_2$ on what FiO$_2$.
- RS: Airway/breath sounds/drains.
- GI: Feeding/aspirate/sounds/drains.
- GU: Input/output/balance.
- Host defence: includes temperature, leucocyte count and microbiology cultures
- Skin: Pressure areas.

INVESTIGATIONS

Not all will be necessary every day. They are grouped together in as logical a manner as possible.

- FBC/U&E/LFT/Ca^+/Mg^+/Amylase/Clotting/D-dimer/Traces/CRP
- CXR/ECG.
- ABG(state FiO_2).
- 24 hr urine/creatinine clearance/osmolalities.
- Microbiology: Hep B status/swabs/sputum/blood cultures/urines/line cultures.
- Pregnancy test: Do not make assumptions about unknown, unconscious female patients.
- Blood products available.
- Blood levels: Theraputic ranges:

Clonazepam	20 - 70 ng/ml
Diazepam	600 - 1200 ng/ml
Digoxin	0.5 - 2.0 ng/ml
Lignocaine	4 - 6 mcg/ml
Lithium	0.5 - 1.3 mmol/l
Phenobarbitone	10 - 25 mcg/ml
Phenytoin	10 - 25 mcg/ml
Theophylline	10 - 20 mcg/ml
Thiocyanate	< 100 mcg/ml
Valproate	50 - 100 mcg/ml

TREATMENT

- IPPV: V_E/Mean airway pressure/FiO_2;CPAP/ASB; Physio
- Sedation/analgesia/paralysis
- Fluids/Feeding ± insulin
- Gastric mucosal protection
- DVT prophylaxis
- Antibiotics (state number of days)
- Inotropic support
- Dialysis

FIRST IMPRESSIONS

WARD ROUND AND PLAN

Persons present on ward round/plan for today/for next few days/ultimate objective/explanation given to relatives.

THERAPEUTIC INTERVENTION SCORING SYSTEM

This is an index of nursing intensity and can be used for costing purposes. It does not indicate severity of condition on admission and neither does it predict outcome. One ITU nurse should be able to manage 40 - 50 TISS points.

4 POINTS	3 POINTS
Cardiac arrest	Total parenteral nutrition
Controlled ventilation	Pacing available
Ventilation with muscle relaxants	Chest drain
Balloon tamponade of varices	Assisted spontaneous respiration
Arterial infusion	Continuous positive airways pressure
Pulmonary artery catheter	KCl infusion
Pacing	Intubated
Haemodialysis (For acute renal failure)	Regular airway suction (no tube)
Peritoneal dialysis	Complex metabolism
Induced hypothermia	Multiple ABG
Infusion requiring pressure bag	Infusion blood products
G-suit	Multiple IV drugs
CO measurement	More than 3 IV lines
Platelet transfusion	Vasoactive drugs
Aortic balloon pump	Arrhythmia infusions
Extra corporeal membrane oxygenation	Cardioversion
Surgery within 24h	Space blanket
Lavage of GI bleed	Arterial line
Emergency endoscopy	Acute digoxin
	Active diuresis
	Correct acidosis/alkalosis
	Emergency paracentesis
	Acute anticoagulation
	Phlebotomy
	More than 2 antibiotics
	Treatment of seizures

2 POINTS	1 POINT
CVP	ECG
2 venous access	Hourly observations
Haemodialysis (For chronic renal failure)	Open IV
Tracheostomy within 24 hours	Anticoagulation
Spontaneous respiration via tube	Standard input/output
Tracheostomy care	Frequent U&E
Acute cannulation	Intermittent IV drugs
Chemotherapy	Multiple dressing changes
	Traction
	IV antimetabolite
	Skin ulcer treatment
	O_2 by facemask or cannulae
	IV antibiotics
	Physiotherapy
	Wound irrigation, packing
	GI decompression

PRACTICALITIES OF VENTILATORS AND VENTILATION

CLASSIFICATION OF VENTILATORS

HUNTER 1961: Divided into volume pre-set and pressure pre-set.
MAPLESON 1962: Flow generated ventilators (FGV) or pressure generated ventilators (PGV)
WARD 1973: Low-powered or high-powered;
1. Mechanical thumbs
2. Minute volume dividers
3. Bag squeezers
4. Intermittent blowers
INSPIRATION: Pressure/time graphs are straight lines with FGV but curves with PGV.
INSPIRATORY-EXPIRATORY CHANGE (CYCLING):
By volume, flow, pressure or time.

EXPIRATION:
Can be passive or assisted.

EXPIRATORY-INSPIRATORY CHANGE:
Can be patient triggered, or by time or by volume, i.e. when bellows are full.

WHEN TO INTUBATE
The commonest reason is to facilitate ventilation. This can be further broken down as follows.
1. To protect the upper airway; shared airway, trauma, unstable fractures;
2. To protect the lower airway; risk of soiling from gastric contents;
3. When paralysis is required for surgery.

WHEN TO VENTILATE
1. Acute respiratory insufficiency or arrest.
2. Respiratory failure refractory to ↑FiO_2 and other measures.
3. Progressive accumulation of CO_2.
4. Mechanical compromise, e.g. flail chest.
5. Intubation, if prolonged

INDICATIONS FOR TRACHEOSTOMY
1. To bypass obstruction above the level of the trachea.
2. To separate passage of food and air.
3. To permit repeated aspiration of secretions.
4. To allow prolonged ventilation.

HOW TO VENTILATE
Start with minimum intervention and increase as necessary, i.e.:
Spontaneous respiration via T-Piece
↓
Continuous Positive Airways Pressure (CPAP)
↓
Biphasic Positive Airways Pressure (BIPAP)
↓
Pressure Support, Assisted Spontaneous Breathing
↓
Intermittent Mandatory Ventilation (IMV, SIMV)
↓
Intermittent Positive Pressure Ventilation
↓ (IPPV)
IPPV with Positive End Expiratory Pressure
(PEEP)

SETTING UP IPPV
1. Set V_T at 10-15 ml/kg
2. Set f at 8-10 /min initially
3. Set V_E so as to achieve PaCO2 in normal range, by adjusting f initially and V_T if necessary
4. Start with FiO_2 at 1.0 and reduce to lowest level that keeps SpO_2 acceptable, i.e. above 90%, adding PEEP as necessary.

ADJUSTMENT OF IPPV
Think of manipulating three parameters:

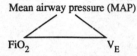

$V_E = V_T \times f$

V_T = inspiratory flow rate x inspiratory time
f = 60 / (inspiratory time + expiratory time)

Mean airway pressure is proportional to:
- Compliance
- PEEP
- I:E ratio - may be reversed

AIR TRAPPING is occurring when auscultation reveals that inspiration is encroaching on expiration. It is a defect due to poor lung compliance and results in defective gas exchange and possibly in barotrauma. The pattern of ventilation will have to be altered.

ADDITION OF PEEP: For example,

FiO₂ 21 30 40 50 60 60 60 60 60 60 70 80 90 100
PEEP 0--0---0---0--0---5--10-15-20-15-15-15-15
                                      ↓↓
                          only for 20 mins
              consider chemically correcting acidosis

HIGH FREQUENCY VENTILATION (HFV)

High frequency ventilation is defined as ventilation at more than four times the normal rate, and requires much smaller tidal volumes (1 - 3 ml/kg). High frequency positive pressure ventilation (HFPPV) is fast IPPV, at 60 - 120 cycles per minute (cpm), via a conventional tube. HF Oscillation depends on a sinusoidal pattern of flow generated by a loudspeaker cone. The Hayak oscillator requires no tube, but uses a cuirass. High frequency jet ventilation (HFJV) is the commonest HFV mode.

HIGH FREQUENCY JET VENTILATION
The equipment consists of the following:
1. High frequency jet ventilator.
2. Mixer unit.
3. O_2 and air sources (both 4 bar).
Portex gas monitoring tube or Mallinkrodt Hi-Lo tube. Some such tubes have two additional lumens, one each for the jet and for sampling.

USES
1. Thoracic and laryngeal surgery.
2. ITU: In acute respiratory distress syndrome and withdrawing ventilation - patient can talk and breathe.
3. Bronchopleural fistula.
4. Bronchoscopy, with Sanders injector.

SETTING UP HFJV
1. Set I:E ratio (as %) 30% (range 10% - 70%).
2. Rate (RR) 150/min (range 40 - 600).
3. Catheter set 3.
4. Driving pressure (Pd) 1.2 - 1.5 bar (max. 3).
5. (Minute volume is calculated by the machine and not measured).
6. FiO_2: the mixer delivers a set oxygen concentration to the jet port. A second line can be connected to the endotracheal tube via a T-piece, in which case the gas entrained is the same as the driving gas. Without a T-piece, room air is entrained into the endotracheal tube, and FiO_2 cannot be measured.

MONITORING HFJV
1. By arterial blood gas analysis. This is the best method, but cannot provide continuous data.
2. Single-breath end-tidal CO_2 using a capnograph and the machine in manual mode.

ADJUSTMENT OF HFJV
- PCO_2: If low, and there is a tendency for this to happen, increase respiratory rate or decrease driving pressure (Pd) this also has the effect of reducing SpO_2, but this can be compensated by then increasing respiratory rate.
- PO_2: If low, and the tendency in normal lungs is for it to rise, increase respiratory rate (which increases PEEP) or increase I:E ratio.

ADVANTAGES OF HFJV
1. Increased cardiovascular stability.
2. Less barotrauma, of benefit to lung and anastomosis.
3. Better operative field.
4. Double lumen tube not required.
5. Possible to operate on a pulmonary lobe without letting down the lung.

DISADVANTAGES OF HFJV
1. Heat loss - the inspired gas can be warmed, but the entrained gas cannot.
2. Moisture loss - a humidifier can be attached via a T-piece at the ventilator, delivering 20 ml/hr of saline.
3. Impossible to use a volatile, requires total intravenous anaesthesia.

WITHDRAWAL OF VENTILATORY SUPPORT

Reversal of cascade, from most interventional to least, checking all parameters in each stage.
1. Reversal of paralysis and reduction of sedation.
2. Change IPPV to SIMV, progressively reducing fIMV, so patient has to take more breaths at a higher threshold.
3. Change SIMV to CPAP, often by increasing periods; may need to ventilate formally overnight, for example.
4. From CPAP onto T-Piece.

WHEN TO EXTUBATE
Is the condition, for which the patient was intubated, better?
Criteria:
1. Cardiovascular and metabolic stability.
2. Protection of airway.
3. $PaO_2 > 7$ kPa on $FiO_2 < 0.4$.
4. Vital Capacity > 15 ml/kg, with ability to increase it voluntarily.
5. Patient can sustain inspiratory pressure in excess of -30cmH$_2$O for 10 seconds.
6. RR/Vt (in litres) < 100.

REPLACEMENT OF DEFECTIVE TRACHEAL TUBE
1. Increase FiO2 to preoxygenate.
2. Laryngoscopy, suction.
3. Pass new tube into pharynx.
4. Cuff leak test; deflate cuff, leak indicates presence of adequate lumen for new tube.
5. Change tube.

CARDIORESPIRATORY MANIPULATION

ACUTE RESPIRATORY DISTRESS SYNDROME: DEFINITION
1. Identifiable acute lung injury.
2. Normal albumin.
3. PCWP <15.
4. Decreased compliance.
5. Increased shunt.
6. Divide PaO_2 (mmHg)/FiO_2: 150-300 implies injury, <150 indicates ARDS.
7. CXR demonstrates bilateral infiltrates.

THE SHOEMAKER GOALS
Some now regard these as trials and not goals; in other words, if the patient's physiology is capable of meeting these targets, the patient is more likely to survive.

CARDIAC INDEX	150% of normal; > 4.5 $l/min/m^2$
DO_2	> 600 ml/min/m^2
VO_2	130% of normal; > 170 ml/min/m^2
BLOOD VOLUME	500 ml more than normal

BIHARI PROTOCOL : OPTIMISING DO_2
1. Volume load: Using blood and 4.5% albumin. Aim for:
- PCWP 16 mmHg
- CVP 12 mmHg
- Hb 12 -15 g/dl
2. Low dose dopamine and dobutamine, in order to keep CI over 4.5 $l/min/m^2$.
3. Adrenaline + noradrenaline, to keep mean arterial pressure over 60 mmHg.
4. Vasodilation: Use prostacyclin, PGI_2 5 - 30 ng/kg/min. However adequate mean pressure is required to allow this.
   $\rightarrow$ increased microcirculatory flow
   $\rightarrow$ platelet inhibition in DIC
(Normal vascular compliance = 330 ml/cmH_2O)

HAEMODYNAMIC DECISION MAKING

Another way of looking at the problem, by knowledge of cardiac index and wedge pressure:

	PAWP < 18	PAWP > 18
CARDIAC INDEX > 2.2	I: NORMALITY: NO ACTION REQUIRED	III: DIURETIC + VASODILATOR
CARDIAC INDEX < 2.2	II: VOLUME	IV: INOTROPIC SUPPORT + VASODILATOR

ANTIBIOTICS ON ITU

SEPSIS SYNDROME

It is important if sepsis is suspected to get a baseline C-reactive protein (CRP), which is a marker of bacterial infection.

Diagnosis is based on:

1. Fever over 38.3°c or hypothermia less than 35.6 °C.
2. Tachycardia greater than 90 bpm.
3. Tachypnoea over 20 bpm or requiring ventilation.
4. Hypotension: Systolic blood pressure less than 90 mmHg or having fallen by 40 mmHg, or two of:

   a. Unexplained metabolic acidosis with BE greater than -5 mmol/l

   b. Acute renal failure with urine output below 0.5 ml/kg/hr

   c. Impaired cognition

   d. Arterial hypoxaemia

   e. Coagulopathy

   f. Cardiac index (CI) over 4.0 with systemic vascular resistance index (SVRI) less than 1400.

The following are suggestions only. Definitive therapy depends on culture and sensitivity. While waiting for this, most units have guidelines for specific situations.

LINE INFECTION; flucloxacillin 0.25 - 1.0 g qds + fucidin 580 mg tds or gentamicin 3 mg/kg od.

INTRA-ABDOMINAL INFECTION; metronidazole 500 mg tds+ cefotaxime 1 - 2 g tds; or, piperacillin 100 - 300 mg/kg/d divided doses + gentamicin.

COMMUNITY ACQUIRED PNEUMONIA; erythromycin 50 mg/kg od + cefuroxime 0.75 - 1.5 g tds; or, amoxycillin 0.5 - 1.0 g tds + fluclox + erythromycin.

NOSOCOMIAL PNEUMONIA; flucloxacillin + cefotaxime

MENINGOCOCCAL SEPTICAEMIA; benzylpenicillin 2.4 g every 4 - 6 hours.

OTHER MENINGITIS; benzylpenicillin + chloramphenicol 50 - 100 mg/kg/d divided doses +/- cefotaxime or gentamicin if septic.

INFECTIVE ENDOCARDITIS; gentamicin + benzylpenicillin or ampicillin, + fluclox if Staph. aureus possible.

NEUTROPENIC PATIENTS; piperacillin + gentamicin + antifungal after 3 days (fluconazole 1 - 2 mg/kg/d).

TOTAL BLIND THERAPY; flucloxacillin + cefotaxime + metronidazole.

SECOND LINE AGENTS
Ceftazidime 1 - 2 g bd
Ciprofloxacin 200 mg bd
Imipenem 1 - 2 g/d divided doses
Teicoplanin 400 mg, then 200 mg/d
Vancomycin 500 mg qds
Aztreonam 1 - 2 g tds
Amphotericin 0.25 - 1.0 mg/kg/d

MANAGEMENT OF ACUTE POISONING

1. RESUSCITATION.
2. CANNULATION and samples to lab for immediate assay of paracetamol and salicylate levels; retain serum for toxicology.
3. HISTORY, from Ambulance crew and relatives. Do not trust the patient.
4. EMPTY STOMACH (not in case of paraffin or corrosive ingestion - risk of aspiration) and instillation of activated charcoal (even in delayed presentation, as it may interrupt enterohepatic circulation of drugs). Leave a nasogastric tube in. Repeated charcoal instillation is useful for drugs with a small volume of distribution but long t½, such as barbiturates, theophylline, digoxin and salicylates.
5. SECONDARY SURVEY: CXR, ABG, catheter, CO level.
6. SPECIFIC ANTIDOTES:

β-blockers	atropine, isoprenaline, glucagon
CO	hyperbaric O_2 (t½ of COHb is 250 min in air, 50 min in 100% O_2, and 22 min at 2.5 bar.)
Cyanide	dicobalt edetate 20 ml i.v. chelates CN, Na thiosulphate 50 ml 25% presents sulphur substrate for enzyme.
Opioids	naloxone
Benzodiazepines	flumazenil
Paracetamol	N-acetylcysteine
Digoxin	Dig-specific Fab antibody fragments (Digibind)
Metals	chelating agents: desferrioxamine, dimercaprol, penicillamine.
Organophosphorus	atropine, oximes, pyridostigmine (used for prophylaxis).
Ethylene glycol	ethanol
Sympathomimetics	β-blockers
Phenothiazines	benztropine
Anticholinergics	physostigmine
Oxidising agents	methylene blue

7. SPECIFIC MEASURES: E.g. pacing in tricyclic toxicity.
8. DIURESIS OR DIALYSIS: Keep urinary pH over 6.5 to prevent myoglobin deposition. Mannitol is better than frusemide. For dialysis to be effective, the toxin must have a small Vdss, and minimal protein binding.

For dialysis, it must be of low molecular weight; for filtration, it must have a high affinity for the adsorbant. There is no point in either measure if the extracorporeal clearance is exceeded by the endogenous clearance of the substance.

PHONE NUMBERS OF POISONS UNITS:
London 0171 635 9191;
Newcastle 0191 232 5131;
Leeds 0113 430715;
Edinburgh 0131 229 2477;
Cardiff 01222 709901;
Belfast 01232 240503.

DIALYSIS

In acute renal failure, urea rises by 5 mmol/l/day and creatinine by 15 µmol/l/day. Most would advocate dialysis at 30 mmol/l urea. Only drugs present in plasma can be eliminated by dialysis, thus they must be water soluble and with a small volume of distribution. Lipid soluble drugs may be eliminated by haemofiltration, allowing longer equilibration between compartments.

PERITONEAL DIALYSIS (PD)
USES: Treatment of acute renal failure (ARF), chronic renal failure (CRF); cooling in hyperpyrexia.
REQUIREMENTS: Insertion of silastic Tenchkoff catheter into peritoneum inferior to the umbilicus in the midline.
METHOD: Instil 1000 ml dialysate with 500u heparin at body temperature (unless hyperpyrexial), dwell 30 minutes, drain over 30 minutes; one cycle = one hour. Composition of dialysate, in terms of osmolality and potassium especially, is dictated by the condition.
ADVANTAGES: Simpler than other modes, better for children. Safer with bleeding problems than other modes. Relatively inexpensive. The most cardiovascularly stable method.
DISADVANTAGES: Slow elimination of toxins and excess fluids, therefore inappropriate in highly catabolic states. Needs intact peritoneum. Relatively contraindicated in ventilated patients, and in respiratory distress. Peritonitis is a risk.

HAEMODIALYSIS (HD)

USES: Treatment of ARF, CRF; elimination of poisons; correction of fluid overload.

REQUIREMENTS: Arterial and large-bore venous access. Dialysis machine which presents the blood to a membrane adjacent to the dialysate (see PD).

METHOD: Formation of shunt (often at wrist) or separate arterial and venous cannulae, priming of machine, heparin infusion 1000 u/hr.

ADVANTAGES: More rapid elimination of toxins and fluid than PD.

DISADVANTAGES: Access, expense, bleeding, aluminium toxicity, removal of vitamins and water-soluble nutrients. Air embolus, haemolysis.

CONTINUOUS ARTERIO-VENOUS HAEMOFILTRATION (CAVH)

USES: Treatment of ARF, CRF; elimination of poisons; correction of fluid overload.

REQUIREMENTS: Arterial and large-bore venous access. Filter.

METHOD: Access, priming of filter, heparin.

ADVANTAGES: No pump required.

DISADVANTAGES: Diverts up to 250 ml/min of cardiac output and may precipitate hypotension and hypoperfusion. Tends to clot if MAP not high enough. Access, bleeding, removal of vitamins and water-soluble nutrients. Air embolus.

CONTINUOUS VENO-VENOUS HAEMOFILTRATION (CVVH)

USES: Treatment of ARF, CRF; elimination of poisons; correction of fluid overload.

REQUIREMENTS: Double large-bore venous access. Blood pump and bubble trap. Filter. No dialysate required.

METHOD: Access, priming pump and filter, heparin.

ADVANTAGES: Does not divert cardiac output.

DISADVANTAGES: Access, expense, bleeding, removal of vitamins and water-soluble nutrients. Air embolus, haemolysis.

HAEMODIAFILTRATION

USES: Treatment of ARF, CRF; elimination of poisons; correction of fluid overload.

REQUIREMENTS: Double large-bore venous access. Blood pump and bubble trap. Filter. Employs countercurrent mechanism exposing dialysate to filter.

METHOD: Access, priming pump and filter, run through dialysate, heparin.

ADVANTAGES: Very efficient. As with veno-venous, no cardiac shunt.

DISADVANTAGES: Access, expense, bleeding, removal of vitamins and water-soluble nutrients. Air embolus, haemolysis.

HAEMOPERFUSION

USES: Elimination of poisons, severe hepatic failure.

REQUIREMENTS: Double large-bore venous access, pump, adsorption circuit (amberlite resin or activated charcoal) and heparin.

METHOD: Access, priming, heparin.

ADVANTAGES: In elimination of lipid-soluble and protein-bound toxins, such as barbiturates, tricyclics, paracetamol, salicylates, paraquat, aminophylline and organophosphorus compounds.

DISADVANTAGES: Access, expense, bleeding, haemolysis, thrombocytopenia. Inappropriate for ARF. Does not remove excess fluid as efficiently as other methods.

PACEMAKERS

Pacemakers are common in elderly patients, who will have ischaemic heart disease.

PACEMAKER CODING
This is presented as a series of 3 or 5 letters; for example, VVI is ventricle paced, ventricle sensed, inhibited.
I: Chamber paced; Ventricle, Atrium, Dual.
II: Chamber sensed; V,A,D, None.
III: Mode of response; Triggered, Inhibited, Dual, None, Reverse.
IV: Programmable functions; P = simple programmable, M = multiprogrammable, C = communicating, 0 = none.
V: Antidysrhythmia function; Bursts, Normal rate competition, Scanning, External.

SUXAMETHONIUM may cause inappropriate inhibition.
DIATHERMY may deprogramme the pacemaker or may set up induced current in the wire if current is parallel to it, destroying the box or injuring the myocardium, increasing the threshold.
MAGNETS, although they may convert VVI to VOO (fixed rate) may also deprogramme sophisticated pacemakers.

TEMPORARY PACING: INDICATIONS
1. Complete heart block.
2. Second degree heart block: symptomatic type I, any type II.
3. Symptomatic first degree block.
4. Trifascicular block; any AV block with two other conduction defects, or alternating RBBB/LBBB.

TEMPORARY PACING: METHOD
Right internal jugular cannulation, with Xray screening for siting of wire, and lignocaine cover if ventricle is irritable. Increase voltage until capture of ventricular contraction occurs, indicating threshold. An initial threshold of < 1 volt at 1 ms pulse width is preferable. Set on double this threshold, check daily for increase.

BRONCHOSCOPY

This is how to record what you have done.

- SET UP: Instrument used/indication.
- PREPARATION: Position/pre-oxygenation/suction/sedation.
- PORTAL: Oral/nasal endotracheal or tracheostomy tube.
- FINDINGS: Trachea/carina/mucosa/main bronchi/bronchus intermedius/lobar bronchi; blood/secretions/plugs/sputum/foreign material.
- PROCEDURE: Lavage/suction/brushings/biopsy.
- POST-PROCEDURE: O_2/ventilation/position.

BRAIN DEATH

This is recognised in the UK as being synonymous with death. There are preconditions which have to be established and exclusions to be considered before the diagnosis can be made on the criteria below.

PRECONDITIONS
1. Apnoeic coma.
2. Irreversible damage of known cause.

EXCLUSIONS
Brain death cannot be diagnosed if any of these exist.
1. Hypothermia below 35°c.
2. Sedative or hypnotic drugs present.
3. Acid-base derangement.
4. Metabolic disorder.
5. Elevated $PaCO_2$
6. Hypotension.

CRITERIA
Performed twice (by convention rather than law) at least 30 min apart, more than 6 hours after the event causing death, by 2 doctors. Neither may be from the transplant team and both must have been registered more than 5 years, one being a consultant.
1. Pupils: direct and consensual responses: tests second cranial nerve (CII) and parasympathetics.
2. Corneal reflex; tests CV & CVII.
3. Pain to face; tests CV & CVII.

4. Doll's eye; in brain stem death, the eyes stay fixed in sockets; this tests CVIII.
5. Caloric test; 30 ml ice cold water applied to clear meatus; no nystagmus implies brain stem death; tests CVIII.
6. Gag; tests CIX & CX.
7. Apnoea; Set FiO_2 to 1.0, then disconnect, continuing to give O_2 via cannulae at 6 l/min. Brain stem death is likely if no effort after 10 min or $PaCO_2$ rises above 6.6 kPa.

THE CORONER

The following must be reported to the Coroner. It is often wise to discuss a postoperative death, or the death of an intensive care patient, with the coroner or his representative in any case:

1. SUDDEN DEATH: Not seen by doctor within 14 days
2. MURDER, SUICIDE
3. DRUGS, POISONS, MEDICAL TREATMENT
4. FACTORY ACCIDENT
5. PENSION: Industrial Disability or War
6. ALCOHOL, SELF NEGLECT
7. INFANT, FOSTER CHILD
8. FOLLOWING ABORTION
9. IN CUSTODY OR PRISON
10. ROAD TRAFFIC ACCIDENT

Resuscitation and critical incident management

CRITICAL INCIDENT RECOGNITION AND MANAGEMENT

All management algorithms commence with basic life support; control of the airway, confirmation of breathing and oxygenation, and support of the circulation. Most then proceed to advanced life support, as follows. Specific measures are listed under each condition. ALL MANAGEMENT PLANS ASSUME THAT BASIC AND ADVANCED LIFE SUPPORT HAVE BEEN INSTITUTED. Failed intubation is covered in the Practical Anaesthesia section; poisoning is covered under Intensive Care.

CARDIAC ARREST

RECOGNITION:
a. Fit, proceeding to immediate unconsciousness.
b. Absent pulses;
   Palpable Carotid = 60 mmHg
   Palpable Femoral = 70 mmHg
   Palpable Radial   = 80 mmHg
c. Ashen cyanosis.
d. Pupillary dilation.
e. Alarming gasping - often obstructed in character.

AIRWAY OBSTRUCTION

RECOGNITION:
a. Cyanosis.
b. Paradoxical chest movement.
c. Tachycardia.

If you can't control an airway, you should be doing something else, like dermatology, perhaps, instead of reading this book.

VF & PULSELESS VT

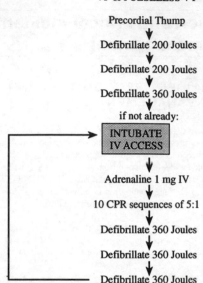

Precordial Thump
↓
Defibrillate 200 Joules
↓
Defibrillate 200 Joules
↓
Defibrillate 360 Joules
↓
if not already:

**INTUBATE
IV ACCESS**
↓
Adrenaline 1 mg IV

10 CPR sequences of 5:1
↓
Defibrillate 360 Joules
↓
Defibrillate 360 Joules
↓
Defibrillate 360 Joules

CONSIDER -DIFFERENT PADDLE POSITIONS;
-DIFFERENT DEFIBRILLATOR;
-OTHER ANTI ARRYTHMIC DRUGS;
-ADRENALINES 5 mg AND
-ALKALISING AGENTS AFTER 3 LOOPS

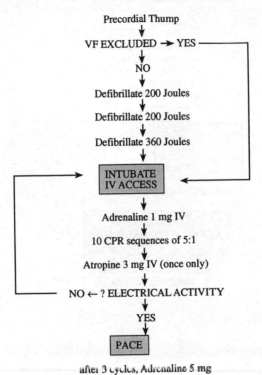

ASYSTOLE

Precordial Thump

↓

VF EXCLUDED → YES ─────────┐

↓

NO

↓

Defibrillate 200 Joules

↓

Defibrillate 200 Joules

↓

Defibrillate 360 Joules

↓

**INTUBATE
IV ACCESS**

↓

Adrenaline 1 mg IV

↓

10 CPR sequences of 5:1

↓

Atropine 3 mg IV (once only)

↓

NO ← ? ELECTRICAL ACTIVITY

↓

YES

↓

PACE

after 3 cycles, Adrenaline 5 mg

ELECTROMECHNICAL DISSOCIATION

EXCLUDE

        Hypovolaemia
        Pneumothorax
        Cardiac tamponade
        Pulmonary embolus
        Overdose
        Hypothermia
        Electrolyte imbalance

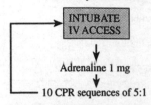

INTUBATE
IV ACCESS

Adrenaline 1 mg

10 CPR sequences of 5:1

CONSIDER;
CALCIUM CHLORIDE 10ml
10%
PRESSOR AGENTS
ALKALINISING AGENTS
ADRENALINE 5mg

MALIGNANT HYPERPYREXIA

RECOGNITION:
a. $\uparrow Ca^{++} \rightarrow$ myofibril ATPase $\rightarrow$ HEAT: $\uparrow 2°C$ per hour
b. $\uparrow Ca^{++} \rightarrow$ troponin-C $\rightarrow$ RIGIDITY
c. $\uparrow Ca^{++} \rightarrow$ phosphorylase kinase $\rightarrow$ GLYCOGENOLYSIS
Beware: Family history, young, squints; and the fact that not all the signs may be present. Capnography is the single most useful monitor. It is possible to have had previous uneventful anaesthesia.

FEATURES:
Affects 3:1 male : female; associated with squints and musculoskeletal abnormalities. Autosomal dominant inherited structural abnormality of sarcolemma or sarcoplasmic reticulum. Incidence is 1:200,000 (UK). Diagnosis is based on muscle biopsy; if contracture of 0.2 g occurs in halothane 2% and caffeine 2 mmol/l, this is malignant hyperpyrexia susceptible (MHS). The patient is MH equivocal (MHE) if one or other. MH non-susceptible (MHN) if neither, but the testing is only 95% sensitive. The condition has a 10% mortality.

There is a ryanodine receptor gene, associated with calcium channels in sarcoplasmic reticulum. This is associated, by no means universally, with chromosome 19 q12 - 13.2.

MANAGEMENT:
1. Stop trigger agent and stop surgery if possible.
2. 100% O_2 .
3. Hyperventilate.
4. Dantrolene (modal effect 2.4 mg/kg, range 1 - 10 mg/kg).
5. Correct acidosis/arrhythmia/hyperkalaemia, encourage diuresis; retain urine for myoglobin assay.
6. Cool.
7. Transfer to ITU and monitor progress of condition by serum CK at 6, 12 and 24 hours.
Morning after diagnosis: Myoglobinuria, and disproportionate rise in plasma CK. Screen proband and family.

ALLERGIC REACTION

RECOGNITION:
a. Cardiovascular: Hypotensive collapse, pulmonary hypertension.
b. Respiratory: Bronchospasm, oedema.
c. Skin: Urticaria, oedema, flushing.
Beware especially: suxamethonium, thiopentone, older neuromuscular blocking agents, and the immediate post-induction period.

DEFINITIONS:
- INTOLERANCE: Qualitatively normal, quantitatively abnormal reaction to drug.
- IDIOSYNCRACY: Qualitatively abnormal, but not immunologically-mediated, response to drug.
- ANAPHYLAXIS: IgE-mast cell histamine release reaction, type I hypersensitivity.
- ANAPHYLACTOID: Direct histamine release from mast cells and macrophages.

MANAGEMENT:
1. Stop administration of suspected agent.
2. 100% O_2.
3. External cardiac massage if no pulse.
4. Adrenaline 0.5 - 1.0 ml of 1:10,000.
5. Nebulised bronchodilators.
6. Chlorpheniramine 10 mg.
7. Steroids.
8. Plasma expansion 70 ml/kg.
9. Aminophylline 250 mg over 5 minutes.

INVESTIGATION: Blood samples into two EDTA bottles at each of 0, 3, 6, 12 and 24 hours after event, store at -25°C, and send to Sheffield.
- Allergy is investigated at Sheffield, 01742 766222
- MH is investigated at Leeds, 0113 433144 Hot line 01345 333111.
- Scoline apnoea is investigated at the RPMS Hammersmith, 0181 743 2030.

AMNIOTIC FLUID EMBOLUS

RECOGNITION: This rare event is said to occur in "turbulent" vaginal delivery, during operative or instrumental delivery, and during abruption.
a.   Dyspnoca.
b.   Cyanosis.
c.   Hypoxaemia.
d.   Hypotension.
e.   Cardiovascular collapse.
f.   Convulsions.
g.   DEATH: AFE carries 80% mortality, which occurs within the first hour.

MANAGEMENT:
1.   This is entirely supportive, and includes, as with all maternal catastrophes:
2.   Immediate delivery of the fetus.

VENOUS AIR EMBOLUS

FEATURES:
a.   During craniotomy, in 2 - 40%.
b.   Sitting position.
c.   Embolus ends in the right ventricle, where it may compromise cardiac output if large enough.
d.   In cases of patent foramen ovale, a paradoxical embolus may occur with return of the embolus to vital tissue which will include the brain.
e.   Nitrous oxide causes any air embolus to enlarge. The use of a stethoscope and a capnograph will allow early detection, with a 'mill wheel' murmur and a decrease in end-tidal CO_2.

MANAGEMENT:
1.   Stop any further embolism by flooding the operation site with saline and packs, and supporting the circulation with 100% oxygen and fluids. Compress neck veins to elevate CVP.
2.   Left side down, elevate legs.
3.   In some cases air may be retrieved from the right side of the heart if a central venous catheter is in place.

STATUS ASTHMATICUS

RECOGNITION:
a. Dyspnoea (inabilty to speak is a grave sign).
b. Cyanosis.
c. Reduced peak expiratory flow rate (PEFR) to less than 30% predicted.
d. Pulsus paradoxus, especially if more than 20 mmHg.
e. Arterial blood gas analysis showing reduced O_2, proceding to hypercapnic (respiratory) acidosis.

Beware: Silent chest, drowsy patient.

MANAGEMENT:
1. Oxygen.
2. Bronchodilators by infusion or nebuliser.
3. Hydrocortisone 4 mg/kg IV.
4. Antibiotics.
5. Ventilation if exhausted or if CO_2 accumulating.

STATUS EPILEPTICUS

RECOGNITION:
a. Tonic-clonic seizures.
b. Cyanosis if intercostals involved.
c. Tongue biting.
d. Incontinence.

MANAGEMENT:
1. Protect from injury.
2. Diazemuls 5 mg/min until seizures controlled. Alternatives include general anaesthesia with thiopentone and a subsequent rapid sequence intubation.

EPIGLOTTITIS

RECOGNITION:
a. Stridor (but this is also seen in croup), and use of accessory muscles.
b. Severe systemic insult (which is not seen in croup).
c. Child aged 3 - 5 (croup is seen between 6/12 months and 3 years).
d. Fever.
e. Drooling.
f. No coryzal signs (contrasting with croup).

MANAGEMENT:
1. Calm atmosphere; avoid moving the child, cannulation or examination; do not lie the child down.
2. Availability of emergency measures for airway control, i.e. tracheostomy.
3. Gaseous induction of anaesthesia, sitting.
4. Intubation; laryngeal opening is where it always is, behind the epiglottis, but the only clue may be bubbles from between the cords.
5. Antibiotics; chloramphenicol and ampicillin.
6. Intubation with or without ventilation for 24 hours.

PROTEINURIC HYPERTENSION (PRE-ECLAMPTIC TOXAEMIA)

Stages:

I	↑BP	Time to onset of crisis: 2 weeks - 3 months
II	↑BP + Proteinuria	Time to onset of crisis: 2 days - 3 weeks
III	↑BP + Proteinuria + Symptoms	Time to onset of crisis: 2 hours - 3 days

IV   Crisis: Eclampsia is seen in 4.9/10,000 births, has a 50% mortality, 44% of whom die in the postpartum period. 42% of cases have no prodrome.

Also: DIC, haemolysis, ARF, ARDS. The HELLP syndrome is haemolysis, elevated liver enzymes, and low platelets.

DIAGNOSTIC INCLUSION CRITERIA: Either A, B or C:

A: Hypertension greater than 150/100 mmHg, plus at least one of:

    Proteinuria more than 0.3g/day.

    Clonus more than 3 beats.

    Symptoms.

    Platelets below 100,000, urate over 0.45 mmol/l, or AST over 30 iu/l.

B: Severe hypertension greater than 170/110 mmHg.

C: Eclampsia.

MANAGEMENT:

VASCULAR ACCESS FBC, Clotting, urate, LFT.

↓

ADMIT LABOUR WARD Catheter +/– invasive monitoring.

↓

INPUT/OUTPUT: BP every 15 min: BLOODS every 12 hours.

Fluid protocol	Anticonvulsant protocol	Antihypertensive protocol	Epidural

↓

(may combine in Mg protocol)

FLUID:

- 1000 ml Hartmann's solution over 12 hours.
- If Hct >0.35, give 500 ml albumin solution.
- If still oliguric with output less than 0.5 ml/kg/hr, institute CVP monitoring.

ANTICONVULSANT: Phenytoin 15 mg/kg (not faster than 50 mg/min) then maintenance 100 mg qds, with ECG monitoring, aiming for plasma level 40-80 µmol/l.

ANTIHYPERTENSIVE: If mean arterial pressure is greater than 125 mmHg, give hydralazine 5 mg repeated every 15 minutes; consider nifedipine 20 mg s/l in refractory cases.

MAGNESIUM:

Magnesium sulphate 4g stat (16 mmol).

Maintenance 1g/hr (4 mmol/hr).

Aim for plasma level 2.0 - 3.5 mmol/l.

Magnesium will depress reflexes and abolish clonus. However in extreme cases it will reduce level of consciousness and muscle tone, and can even cause respiratory embarrassment.

TOTAL SPINAL ANAESTHESIA

RECOGNITION:

a. Rapidly ascending dense block following apparent epidural administration of local anaesthetic. It may also occur in regional blocks around the head and neck.

b. Inability to cough (inspiration is a diaphragmatic movement and thus an unreliable sign, whereas expiration is intercostal).

c. Arm weakness.

d. Loss of consciousness.

e. Cardiovascular collapse as cardiac accelerator fibres (upper thoracic) are blocked, in addition to existing sympathetic block.

MANAGEMENT:

1. Protect airway - intubation will be necessary, but first

2. Administer 100% oxygen.

3. Elevate feet, uterine displacement in the obstetric patient if not delivered.

4. Rapid iv infusion.

5. Vasopressor - ephedrine 6 mg repeated until effect obtained.

6. Ensure prevention of awareness.

MAJOR HAEMORRHAGE

RECOGNITION:
a. Tachycardia, which precedes
b. Hypotension (unless cardiac drugs present).
c. Pallor.
d. Sweating.
e. Cyanosis.
f. Hyperventilation.
g. Confusion.
h. Oliguria.

MANAGEMENT:
1. Resuscitate - see introduction to this section.
2. Multiple wide-bore cannulation and infusion, blood, starches, colloid all probably better than crystalloid. Hypertonic saline is sometimes available.
3. Remember to send for the blood.
4. Pneumatic anti-shock garments.
5. Correct acidosis, electrolyte disturbance and coagulation derangement, if present.
6. Inotropic support to prevent renal failure.

PNEUMOTHORAX

RECOGNITION:
a. Be aware of the risk in trauma, central cannulation, brachial plexus block, during positive pressure ventilation, emphysema, in Marfan's and other tall young men.
b. Cyanosis, tachypnoea.
c. Assymetrical chest movement.
d. Tracheal deviation - away from the side of a tension pneumothorax, towards the side of a simple pneumothorax.
e. Tachycardia and hypotension.
f. Surgical emphysema.

MANAGEMENT:
1. Secure airway.
2. Discontinue nitrous oxide (if in use) and give 100% oxygen.
3. If under tension: 14G cannula into 2nd. intercostal space in mid-clavicular line, prior to
4. Definitive intrapleural drainage.

AWARENESS

Awareness is a major cause of litigation and is seen in paralysed patients (notably when using total intravenous anaesthesia) and obstetrics.

RECOGNITION:
a. Pressure, rate, sweat and tears scale (PRST): Score less than 4 implies sleep.

Systolic BP	<+15	0	Sweat	+/-	0
	<+30	1		+	1
	>+30	2		++	2
Heart Rate	<+15	0	Tears	+/-	0
	<+30	1		+	1
	>+30	2		++	2

b. Isolated forearm technique.
c. Skin conductance.
d. Lower oesophageal sphincter contractility.
e. Frontalis EMG.
f. EEG: awake = low amplitaude, high frequency
asleep = high amplitude, low frequency.
g. Evoked responses: Probably the way forward; auditory or visual.

MANAGEMENT:
1. Avoid it: use a volatile and a volatile monitor.
2. Ensure analgesia and patient safety.
3. Suspend surgery.
4. Full explanation to patient.

POST-TONSILLECTOMY HAEMORRHAGE

RECOGNITION:
a. Irritable child in first 12 hours post tonsillectomy.
b. Hypovolaemia.
c. Occult bleeding, swallowed into stomach, and vomiting.

MANAGEMENT
1. Inhalational induction, or
2. Rapid sequence induction; either way anticipate difficulty and expect to use a smaller tube than at original operation.
3. Extubate awake and on side, head down. The child will vomit.

DIABETIC KETOACIDOSIS

RECOGNITION:
a. Reduced conscious level.
b. Ketones on breath and in urine.
c. Advanced dehydration.
d. Acidosis with increased anion gap.

MANAGEMENT:
1. Insulin by infusion.
2. Correction of hypovolaemia with saline, not dextrose until blood glucose in normal range; up to 100 ml/kg may be required in the initial phase in extreme cases.
3. Attention to serum potassium which will fall with correction of glucose.
4. Use bicarbonate only in extreme cases.

ADDISONIAN CRISIS

RECOGNITION:
a. Apathy, coma.
b. Hypoglycaemia.
c. Hyperkalaemia.
d. Trauma, infection, abrupt withdrawal of steroid therapy, Waterhouse-Friderichsen syndrome.

Beware: Surgical and anaesthetic trauma in the long-term or recent short-term steroid user.

MANAGEMENT:
1. Correction of hypovolaemia.
2. Steroids; both glucocorticoid replacement (hydrocortisone) and mineralocorticoid replacement (fludrocortisone) will be needed.
3. Correction of hyperkalaemia and hyponatraemia.

PULMONARY EMBOLUS

RECOGNITION:
a. Dyspnoea, tachypnoea.
b. Cyanosis.
c. Circulatory collapse.
d. RH strain or S_I Q_{III} T_{III} on ECG.
e. ABG: $\downarrow O_2$ and $\downarrow CO_2$.

Beware: 10th day postop total hip replacement.

MANAGEMENT:
1. Anticoagulation, or in extreme cases:
2. Thrombolysis.
3. Analgesia.
4. Thoracotomy and embolectomy under bypass in refractory situations.

NEONATAL PYLORIC STENOSIS

FEATURES:

a. Obstruction between stomach and duodenum and mismatched loss of electrolyte and buffer from those two sites.

b. The overriding need to conserve Na^+ in the kidneys which prevents correction of the problem.

c. So, while there is vomiting loss of K^+ and H^+, these ions are still excreted in the urine in order to maintain Na^+. The result of this is:

d. Hypochloraemic alkalosis.

e. Hypokalaemia.

f. Haemoconcentration.

MANAGEMENT:

1. Achieve normovolaemia with saline, with potassium supplements. Use Cl- as guide to success in correction of dehydration and acidosis (see page 28).

2. Pass nasogastric tube.

3. Rapid sequence induction after aspiration of tube.

4. Extubate awake following NG aspiration.

5. Infiltrate wound with local anaesthetic.

6. Feed on 2nd. day.

Index